TMJ
SYNDROME
The Overlooked Diagnosis

A. Richard Goldman, D.D.S.
with Virginia McCullough

A FIRESIDE BOOK
Published by Simon & Schuster Inc.
New York   London   Toronto   Sydney   Tokyo

Fireside
Simon & Schuster Building
Rockefeller Center
1230 Avenue of the Americas
New York, New York 10020

First Fireside Edition, 1989

Published by arrangement with Congdon & Weed, Inc.
FIRESIDE and colophon are registered trademarks
of Simon & Schuster Inc.
Manufactured in the United States of America

1   3   5   7   9   10   8   6   4   2   Pbk.

Library of Congress Cataloging in Publication Data
Goldman, A. Richard.
TMJ syndrome: the overlooked diagnosis/A. Richard Goldman, with
Virginia McCullough.—1st Fireside ed.
p.   cm.
Reprint. Originally published: New York: Contemporary Books,
1987.
"A Fireside book."
Includes index.
1. Temporomandibular joint—Diseases.   I. McCullough, Virginia.
II. Title.
RK470.G65   1989
617'.522—dc19   89-1058
CIP
ISBN 0-671-65966-9

Contents

*To those who are chronic pain sufferers with
the hope that they will seek proper help
and, with relief of their problems,
go on to re-create their lives*

Acknowledgments

Many people had a role in shaping my career and, hence, this book. I'd most certainly like to thank my parents, who had the wisdom to encourage my participation in projects that nurtured, rather than stifled, creativity and curiosity.

I am also grateful to a high school chemistry teacher who taught me to ask the following question when faced with an unknown: "What, why, and according to whom?" This teacher also taught me that every question or problem can be looked at in multiple ways.

I've had the opportunity to study with many wonderful clinicians, researchers, and teachers over the years, and I'd like to thank all of them for giving so freely of their knowledge, findings, and selves during the formative part of my professional life.

Few were more encouraging to me than my patients and office staff when the possibility of a book was mentioned. They helped me turn the possibility into a reality. I will always be grateful.

I'd also like to thank Libby McGreevy at Congdon & Weed for her editorial help and her patience.

My wife and two children encouraged me to write this book and were willing to put up with my preoccupation during the long stretches of time in which it was written. I'd also like to thank them for their many sacrifices while I was studying and developing the techniques discussed. I will always be grateful to them for bearing with me during this time.

A. Richard Goldman, D.D.S.

Preface

I've been interested in the diagnosis, treatment, and study of temporomandibular joint dysfunction (TMJ) for almost twenty years. The curiosity I developed about the subject came out of my interest in restorative and reconstructive dentistry. This area of dentistry not only uses advanced concepts of mouth restoration, it also deals with the specifics of how teeth fit together in all their complexities.

After graduating from dental school I began an extensive continuing education program and worked with people all over the country who were directly involved in research and development of various techniques in reconstructive dentistry. This study was done both in their offices and in intensive courses given throughout the country.

When I began to incorporate these techniques into my practice, I noticed that patients who came back for checkups often commented about changes that appeared unrelated to the treatments they had received. "Ever since you made those bridges," one woman said, "my ear problems have cleared up." Another patient said, "Ever since I had the crowns replaced, my headaches are gone." I also began to pay more attention to patients' complaints and was more open to the possibility that dental work could trigger problems.

In the late 1960s, when patients were making these comments, TMJ was little known or recognized, even by dentists. However, a few dentists were beginning to study and attempting to treat TMJ. It became apparent to me that TMJ and reconstructive dentistry were related fields and that the knowledge from each could be combined to develop successful TMJ treatment. Even though little was known about TMJ, I believed that it was a problem with an answer; it was simply a matter of working persistently enough to find that answer.

Also at that time success rates, using the techniques developed, were far less than 50 percent. That still left the majority of TMJ patients suffering. Even today, paltry success rates are common and ignorance and confusion about TMJ abounds.

The present state of confusion about TMJ, on the part of both the general public and health care community, prompted me to start the Institute for the Study and Treatment of Headaches and Facial Pain. The institute created a vehicle by which my colleagues in all branches of health care can learn more about TMJ. It also created a vehicle to educate other dentists about the dental treatment requirements of ex-TMJ patients. If this treatment is done incorrectly, the patient's symptoms are much more likely to return. Because the concept of this treatment isn't available through standard dental education, the institute offers programs to fill this need.

But, first and foremost, the institute is a treatment center for those suffering with TMJ. Treating patients for TMJ problems can be frustrating and personally painful. Patients I see have lived in severe pain—sometimes for many years. They had been unable to seek help in appropriate places because they didn't know about TMJ. Patients spent enormous amounts of money and suffered years of anguish while they looked for help. Many ended up hopeless. This tragic situation prompted me to write this book. Clearly, the public desperately needs education about TMJ—the multitude of symptoms and the potential for cure.

I hope that people who are experiencing some of the difficulties described in this book will talk to their health care providers about TMJ. I hope health care professionals will then be encouraged to learn more about TMJ and the treatment concepts discussed in this book. Through the institute, I would like to share my knowledge and treatment protocol with interested practitioners in all the healing arts.

Today many patients are allowed to continue living in chronic pain simply because information about TMJ is lacking. I hope the institute and this book will contribute to ending this frustrating and often tragic situation.

Note: This book explores the symptoms, causes, and treatment for a specific disorder. The book is not a substitute for seeking appropriate help for persisting symptoms. The people mentioned are actual patients, but their names and other details have been changed.

Introduction

by Alan R. Hirsch, M.D.

What do Thomas Jefferson, Sigmund Freud, Karl Marx, Julius Caesar, Edgar Allen Poe, Lewis Carroll, Charles Darwin, George Bernard Shaw, and thirty million Americans have in common? They all suffer or suffered from recurrent, debilitating headaches. Headaches are ubiquitous in society.

Historically, the treatment of headaches is quite interesting, if not bizarre. Early therapy from old Irish manuscripts instructed the headache sufferer to pray to the eye of Isaiah, the tongue of Solomon, the mind of Benjamin, the heart of St. Paul, and the faith of Abraham. One early therapy involved placing the skins of reptiles over the face and head. Another suggestion was that leeches should be attached to the body to induce bleeding and blister formation on the skin. Still another treatment included the use of seeds from the elder tree, cow's brain and goat dung, all dissolved in vinegar. And yet another early therapy even involved the use of beaver testes bottled in spirits.

There are numerous types of headaches. Some recur and are very painful, yet pose no significant threat to the patient, while others indicate a serious disease. Fortunately, the great majority of headaches fall into the first, or benign, category. Among the more common types of this kind of headache are migraine, cluster, sinus, allergy, chemical sensitivity, and muscle contraction or "tension" headaches. It is to sufferers of these muscle contraction-type headaches (constituting a large portion of the benign category) that Dr. Goldman addresses this book.

Generally, headache pain has more than one cause in a given patient at a given time. Because of the similarities of the types of pain that these different causes can create, the diagnostic challenge is great. Temporomandibular joint dysfunction syndrome must be included as a possible cause (or one of the combination of possible causes) for all headaches.

In *TMJ Syndrome,* Dr. Goldman has eloquently described temporomandibular joint dysfunction. Throughout medical school, this syndrome is barely touched on— perhaps covered in only a single lecture. Yet clearly millions of people suffer from this disease.

Throughout the many years I have seen patients suffering from headache and temporomandibular joint dysfunction, the number who have undergone ineffective treatment and invasive surgical management for their pain has been enormous. I have seen patients who have had all of their teeth removed; people who have had multiple operations on their jaws to alleviate TMJ syndrome. Usually, these approaches have been unsuccessful and have required further treatment.

Dr. Goldman's well thought of and conservative approach to temporomandibular joint dysfunction makes medical sense and has been successful for thousands of patients. His thoughtful and innovative style has assured the diagnosis and successful treatment of temporomandibular joint problems and has also led to the diagnosis of diseases that mimic temporomandibular joint dysfunction. Clearly, Dr. Goldman is to be commended as an example for all of us in the medical community who deal with headache and temporomandibular joint pain.

Alan R. Hirsch, M.D.
Neurologist, Director Hirsch Headache Center
Chicago, Illinois

1

A Dismal Headache

I can't begin to describe the pain. It's simply unbearable.
—a 46-year-old lawyer

"I'm seeing you as a last resort," said Sarah Johnson, a 42-year-old mother of two and former teacher. "When I first began to get regular headaches, I thought they would eventually pass—like a bad cold that seems to hang on and on, but if you wait long enough it finally goes away. But at some point my patience ran out. I was living in constant pain, and I was scared."

To find relief for her headaches, Ms. Johnson took a logical first step. She made an appointment with her family physician and told him her story. "At that point I was having headaches three times a week—big headaches," she explains. When a headache was at its peak, she could do nothing but lie motionless in a dark room. The slightest noise made her flinch. She was completely unavailable to her family and friends until the attack passed.

When her doctor asked her to list any other important symptoms or complaints, she added bouts with stiffness and pain in her neck and shoulders, stuffiness in her ears, and occasional earaches. She also experienced lower back pain

1

much of the time, but had been told there was nothing structurally wrong with her back and so learned to live with some discomfort. Ms. Johnson also reported that her husband often commented (and sometimes complained) that she ground her teeth at night. Not surprisingly, she said her symptoms were worst during times of stress. In times of relative calm, she had some headaches, but they were milder.

The family physician couldn't find any physical cause for Ms. Johnson's headaches, but he did give her a pain reliever to try. He also told her to come back if her problems continued. She returned to his office ten days later. "The pain killer barely dented the pain," she said. Her physician decided it was time to bring in specialists to help solve the puzzle.

Two weeks later Ms. Johnson was in the office of a specialist in diseases of the ears, nose, throat, and sinuses. After a thorough examination, the specialist pronounced her healthy. However, Ms. Johnson observes, "It's difficult to feel healthy when you're walking around in pain."

Although she was discouraged, Ms. Johnson agreed to try a neurologist. She not only had another thorough examination, she also had a CAT scan and an electroencephalogram (EEG). Again she heard discouraging news— no cause, no cure. "And I didn't like the sound of the diagnosis. The neurologist said the headaches appeared to be caused by 'nerves.' "

After months of investigation into her problem of severe, debilitating headaches, Ms. Johnson had:

- A prescription for Valium for her "nerves"
- A narcotic pain reliever
- A referral to a psychotherapist
- Instructions to learn how to manage stress

Ms. Johnson was showing obvious side effects of the pain medication. She had difficulty concentrating, appeared to be tired, and sometimes slurred her words. She concluded her story by saying:

In some ways the medication has helped. I still have the headaches, but when I take the pain killer, the excruciating pain lessens just enough for me not to care about the discomfort. Unfortunately, I don't care about much else either—I really don't function normally, as you no doubt have noticed. My husband had to talk me into keeping today's appointment because I felt so lethargic and 'spacy.' I've been told that I'm nervous and tense. Now the psychotherapist tells me I'm depressed. Of course I'm depressed. It's hard not to be depressed after what I've been through. I was never nervous or tense before, either. But I can't tell you how many hours I've spent worrying about myself. Am I really crazy? Am I imagining all this? Is there a disease the doctors have missed or aren't telling me about? I'm so tired if existing like this. I want my life back.

Ms. Johnson's story may sound bizarre. But it isn't the least bit bizarre or even unusual. I hear variations on the same story every day. Fortunately Ms. Johnson's story has a happy ending. Her condition was properly diagnosed as temporomandibular joint dysfunction syndrome (TMJ). Then an effective treatment plan was developed. (Chapter 10 will explain what this treatment is like.) Today Ms. Johnson has her life back and is living pain-free. She is also teaching school again.

IDENTIFYING TMJ

What is TMJ? Simply put, it is a pain syndrome that leads to some or all of the following symptoms:

- Headaches
- Aching or stiff neck
- Aching or stiff shoulders
- Backaches
- Earaches, ear fullness, ringing in the ears, or pain associated with the ears
- Jaw pain

- Popping or clicking in the jaw joint
- Facial pain
- Numbness in the fingers and toes
- Vertigo (dizziness)
- Undiagnosable tooth pain

These symptoms are caused by spasms, or charley horses, in the muscles of the head, neck, shoulders, and back. The spasms are triggered by a gearing conflict in the teeth. This gearing problem is unrelated to how the teeth look.

By far the most common symptom is headache. Usually, but not always, it is the severity of headaches that drives a person to seek help. But the patient typically experiences other symptoms as well. The severity of symptoms often varies. A person may experience severe headaches, but only mild neck stiffness or backache. A few patients have some of the other symptoms but no headaches at all.

LOOKING FOR RELIEF

If you are a headache sufferer or frequently experience any of the other symptoms, you may have sought help from numerous medical specialists. Depending on your symptoms, you may have been under the care of a chiropractor, a naprapath, or a massage therapist. Many people will obtain some relief for short periods of time. But when the symptoms return, the frustration and anguish mount.

Some undiagnosed TMJ sufferers, particularly those who experience debilitating headaches that prevent any semblance of normal life, may use potent pain relievers. While this therapy will sometimes relieve the pain, a patient may become physically or psychologically addicted to the medication. Even though this kind of therapy rarely helps the TMJ sufferer, extreme discomfort and hope lead the person to continue the treatment.

People who live with chronic pain often become depressed. As they travel futilely from specialist to specialist, they may become more depressed. Eventually many people are referred to psychotherapists for their depression. Ironically, they are then told they probably suffer from headaches because they are depressed! Eventually many people lose hope; some even attempt suicide.

Rarely does TMJ lead people to anything as extreme as suicide. But they may try so hard to help themselves that they feel defeated and helpless. This is particularly common in people who attempt to cope with TMJ symptoms by using various stress-management techniques. While stress affects TMJ's symptoms, the ultimate cause is physiological—a tooth-gearing problem.

OVERCOMING SELF-DEFEAT

Barry Stern had no doubt that in some way he was the cause of his own symptoms. "I've taken up every self-improvement program in the book," he said while giving his history. He had been suffering for about two years before he sought professional evaluation and help. His main symptoms were neck and back stiffness and pain, although he later experienced numbness in his extremities and buzzing in his ears.

Because Mr. Stern attributed his muscle aches and stiffness to stress, he began a vigorous exercise program. "The jogging I did helped me in many ways," he said. "In fact, it became almost like an addiction. I felt more relaxed, but the neck and shoulder pain didn't get better. Sometimes it got worse, but I kept running anyway."

While in training for a marathon, Mr. Stern began to experience numbness in his extremities and later buzzing in his ears. At that point he was also practicing meditation and still believed that all his symptoms were caused by life pressures that he didn't handle well enough. He might have gone on believing that indefinitely if he hadn't mentioned these problems to a physician specializing in sports injuries, whom he was consulting for ankle problems. The sports medicine physician referred him to a neurologist, who gave him a thorough examination and, finding nothing wrong, referred him for TMJ evaluation.

"I'm glad to know I don't have neurological problems," said Mr. Stern, "but I've just about run out of hope about learning how to handle all these strange symptoms. I guess I don't handle life as well as I should."

Mr. Stern's treatment took about eight months, and all his symptoms are gone today. He also was relieved of the self-defeating belief that he brought the pain on himself by being too weak to cope with day-to-day pressures.

You may be a person who has lost, or all but lost, hope of getting any relief from chronic pain. You may also experience guilt over having the symptoms at all. Many patients feel like failures and believe they are weak. I can't offer you guarantees. I wish I could. But I can tell you about TMJ and what can now be done to correct the problem. This book will explain the condition and lead you through an explanation of the symptoms, the diagnosis, and the treatment.

First, it's important to understand the reasons that underlie this often baffling pain syndrome.

2
What Is TMJ?

I thought everybody had a stiff neck and sore shoulders by three in the afternoon! —a 38-year-old salesman

I can't believe the source of all this pain is in my mouth. —a 50-year-old singer

Temporomandibular joint dysfunction syndrome (TMJ) is the name given to an array of symptoms, the majority of which are related to muscle spasms. The muscles involved in the spasms are those which control the movement of the lower jaw. Because we walk on two legs instead of four, these muscles also balance the head, neck, and shoulders.

Why do these muscles go into spasm, with disturbing and sometimes debilitating consequences? The easiest way to explain the reasons for the dysfunction is to describe the normal workings of the jaw and the temporomandibular joint.

BONES AND MUSCLES

Your upper teeth are connected rigidly to your skull. Slightly in front of your ears, on your skull, is a specially shaped bone called the temporal bone. The lower jaw, which is called the mandible, is a horseshoe-shaped bone;

7

its free ends rise upward and end in structures called condyles (see Figure 1). The joint between the temporal bone of the skull and the condyles of the mandible is called the temporomandibular joint (see Figure 2).

If you put your fingers in your ears, press forward, and open and close your mouth, you can feel the condyle move. When you open your mouth, only the lower jaw moves. You can see this for yourself when you look in the mirror and open and close your mouth.

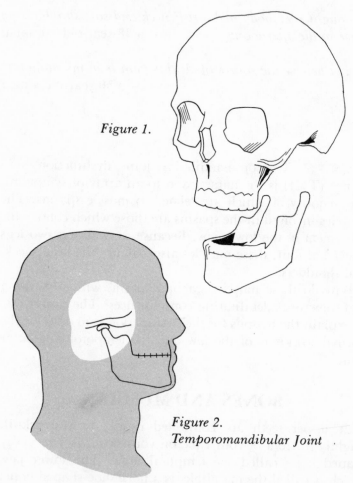

Figure 1.

Figure 2.
Temporomandibular Joint

MOVEMENT IN THE JOINT

Although you have a temporomandibular joint on each side of your head, the two condyles directly affect each other's movement. The reason is that the lower jaw rigidly connects them. When we talk about movement in the joint, we refer to movement occurring on both sides.

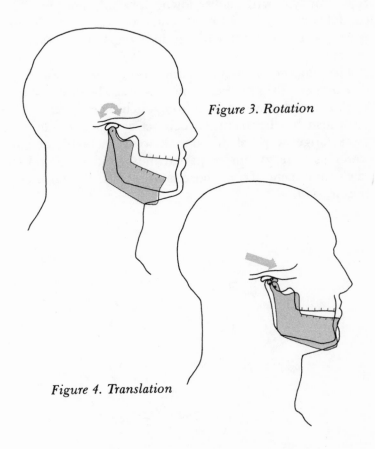

Figure 3. Rotation

Figure 4. Translation

The temporomandibular joint produces two kinds of movement. It can rotate, making a movement like a door hinge (see Figure 3). It can also translate, that is, slide smoothly, much like a ski gliding across the snow (see Figure 4).

The condyle can translate and rotate at the same time. When you begin to open your mouth, the condyle rotates for a very short time. After the initial rotation, it translates forward. Because the condyles are connected by the jawbone, a side-to-side movement produces motion on both sides (see Figure 5). If you move your jaw to the left, the right condyle will move down, forward, and in. The condyle on the left will rotate and move outward. Moving your jaw to the right will produce the same motions in reverse.

The temporomandibular joint has a protective cartilage disc between the upper and lower bones. The disc cushions the bones and prevents them from touching each other. The joint also has ligaments, which act as wires to limit the jaw's range range of motion. Between the skull and the lower jaw are groups of paired muscles that control the jaw's movement. These muscles are called the *muscles of mastication.*

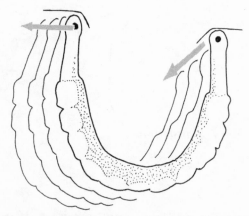

Figure 5. Movement of the Entire Mandible

MUSCLE GROUPS

To give the whole picture, it's necessary to describe these muscle groups and their location. We speak of a muscle in the singular, but remember that each of these has a twin on the other side of the head.

Three pairs of muscles are mainly responsible for closing the mouth. These are the temporalis, the masseter, and the medial pterygoid (see Figures 6, 7, 8). To open the mouth, mylohyoid and digastric muscles work through a chain of other muscles to pull the lower jaw down.

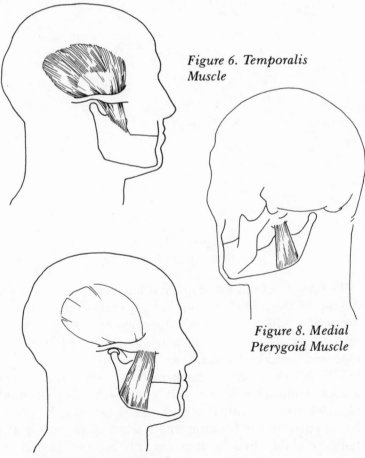

Figure 6. Temporalis
Muscle

Figure 8. Medial
Pterygoid Muscle

Figure 7. Masseter Muscle

The small lateral pterygoids are located deep within the jaw (see Figure 9). Although they have one name, they are actually two muscles originating from the same bone in the skull. One of these muscles connects to the condyle, and as the muscle contracts it pulls the condyle forward. Because of the various restricting ligaments, contraction of the muscle moves the jaw open. The second of the external pterygoids is connected to the disc, and its main purpose is to position the disc when the jaw is closed.

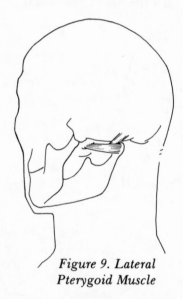

*Figure 9. Lateral
Pterygoid Muscle*

The skull and jaw mechanism is balanced precariously at the top of the spinal column. The spinal column rests on the pelvis, which is in turn supported by the legs. At the upper part of the body, the arms are supported by the rib cage and shoulder complex (see Figure 10).

The muscles connect bone to bone over joints. When muscles contract—shorten their length—they flex the joint. Muscles have no ability to push. They can only be pulled back to their normal resting length when other muscles flex the joint in the opposite direction. The muscles that do this are usually on the other side of the joint (see Figure 11).

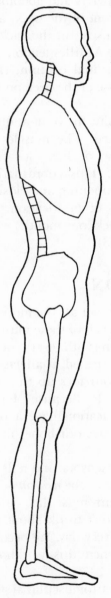

Figure 10. Skeleton

FLEXED MUSCLE

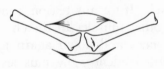

EXTENDED MUSCLE

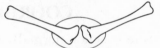

BONES MEETING AT JOINT

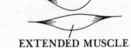

FLEXION

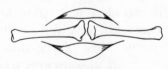

EXTENSION
Figure 11.

In the front of the body, the muscles extend from the toes, up the front of the legs, through the pelvis and abdomen, up to the ribs and shoulders, to the front of the neck, and then connect to the lower jaw. The muscles in the back of the body go from the heel through the Achilles tendon, up the back of the legs, the pelvis, the spinal column, ribs, shoulders, and finally end up at the base of the neck on the skull (see Figure 12).

For us to stand upright, the muscles in the front and the back of the body must be coordinated. The muscles of mastication assume this job because of their location between the front and back muscles. This coordination function is in addition to their job of opening and closing the jaw. Were it not for the muscles of mastication, we would walk with our heads thrown back, our mouths wide open, looking at the sky (see Figure 13).

COORDINATION

For us to function normally and carry out all the motions and activities we engage in every day, each of these muscles must work in a coordinated fashion with every other muscle. If for any reason a muscle is stressed, it affects all the other muscles in the chain from our toes up through our jaws and down again to our heels. Because of this interdependency, the muscles of mastication have a profound effect on our posture and the ways our bones move (see Figure 14).

Our muscle system, plus the nerves, sensors, and reflexes that control it, are given a collective name: the *neuromuscular system*. Most of the time, the neuromuscular system works on an unconscious level. We don't think about the millions of movements we carry out every day. We become conscious of our movements only when this workhorse system needs to protect itself.

Like most systems in the body, the neuromuscular system possesses a marvelous ability to take care of itself, or at least minimize damage. Consider what happens when you walk

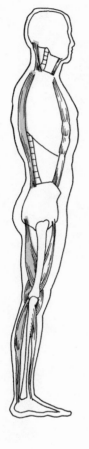

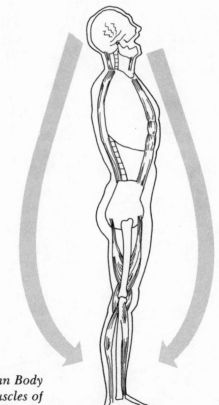

Figure 12. Front and Back
Muscles of the Skeleton

Figure 13. Human Body
Without *the Muscles of
Mastication*

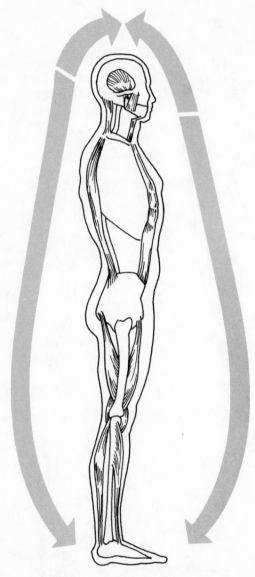

Figure 14. The muscles of mastication are responsible for coordinating the front and back muscles, allowing the body to stand upright.

down the street, step off a curb, and twist your ankle. You may be conscious of pain. Usually you are able to regain your balance and composure and keep on walking. But if the twist was severe enough, you may limp. The limp is the neuromuscular system's way of protecting a potentially injured component.

The neuromuscular system protects itself by using muscles that normally have other functions, as well as changing normal patterns of muscle contraction. We attempt to avoid further injury by this unconscious mechanism. (Athletes and dancers often overextend their bodies and play or perform despite injuries. They sometimes suffer severe consequences by bypassing nature's protective system.)

The limp is an example of the way muscular activity in a leg will follow a repeatable pattern. Because of each muscle's dependence on the whole group, this pattern—in this case a limp—will create a corresponding change in movement patterns in all the other muscles interconnected to it in the chain.

Usually our injuries are slight. The pain of a twisted ankle is gone in a day or two. But if an injury is severe and we limp for a long time, then other muscular problems such as backache are likely to occur.

A SPECIAL JOINT

Muscles are muscles. The muscles of mastication are no different from any others. However, the temporomandibular joint is different from all other joints in its ability to rotate and slide. Even more significant, it has a set of gears connected to it, and each of its parts is forced to mesh. The gears are teeth or tooth replacements such as dentures. You may not think of your teeth as gears, but that's exactly their function in this mechanism.

The teeth, the structures that surround them, and the temporomandibular joint contain sensors for the neuromuscular system. These sensors program the way the jaw moves, similar to the way a computer program will determine how the computer functions.

If there is any abnormality, the neuromuscular system will try to defend the jaw, teeth, and muscles from injury. A common abnormality is a gearing problem between the teeth and the temporomandibular joint (see Figure 15). If a gearing problem exists, then the neuromuscular system programs reflex movements for the lower jaw to help minimize damage to the teeth, their supporting structures, and the temporomandibular joint. This creates a situation in which the jaw is "limping," much as we limp with an injured ankle.

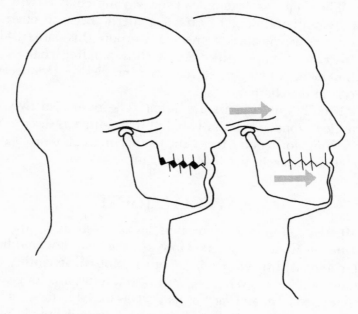

Figure 15. Tooth-Gearing Discrepancy

REBELLION

If life were perfect, the jaw could go merrily along protecting itself. All the other muscles would adjust and compensate for the compensation already being made by the muscles of mastication. This is the way it usually happens. Most people are able to get along quite well. But unfortunately, muscles can sometimes be unforgiving of being pushed beyond their normal physiologic limits for any length of time.

The most common way for a muscle to rebel is to go into spasm—what we sometimes call a charley horse. This condition is a painful contraction of the muscle. One side effect of a muscle spasm is that it sends a message back to the central nervous system. The central nervous system then interprets this signal and causes the muscle in spasm to contract even more.

Now the problem is more than the triggering effect of a tooth-gearing problem. The spasm itself has caused a problem: more painful contraction. When a muscle is in spasm, its change in motion may affect other muscles. The muscle spasm, through the central nervous system, creates more contraction, which then creates more spasm, and this cycle goes on and on (see Figure 16). Because the muscles of mastication coordinate muscles of the back and front of the body, any changes in these muscles can result in postural problems and spasms elsewhere.

Now that you understand how the body supports, balances, and protects itself, it's easy to see the cause of some of the symptoms of TMJ. Because the muscles of mastication are on the head, spasms in these muscles may result in headaches.

Pain can be, and often is, referred to other areas. Referred pain is pain experienced in an area away from the actual cause. Referred pain can be bizarre and may appear to be unfounded.

If the muscle spasms happen to be in one of the muscles that connect the skull to the spinal column and shoulders,

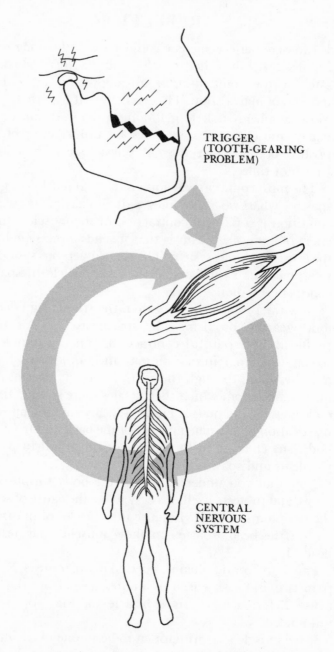

TRIGGER
(TOOTH-GEARING
PROBLEM)

CENTRAL
NERVOUS
SYSTEM

Figure 16. Muscle Spasm Feedback Cycle

this may result in aching, stiffness, and restricted movements in the neck and shoulders. Any muscle that is forced to change its normal range of motion has the potential to go into spasm. This is true of the entire chain. Thus, we see back pain or stiffness in TMJ patients. We even see, although rarely, TMJ symptoms exhibited in the hamstring muscles and in the calves.

Muscle pain may make sense. But why, you ask, would some patients with TMJ have symptoms such as ringing or buzzing in the ears, earaches, dizziness, or even altered hearing? A little muscle called tensor veli palatini is responsible. This muscle has many duties, one of which is to close off the eustachian tubes. The eustachian tubes connect the throat to the middle ear and are responsible for making air pressure in the closed chamber of the middle ear equal to air pressure outside. This occurrence is rarely noticeable. You probably do notice your eustachian tubes at work when you clear your ears during an elevator ride or in flight.

The tensor veli palatini muscle gets its signal from a branch of the same nerve that supplies the external pterygoid muscle, one of the chief muscles involved in TMJ. When the external pterygoid muscle goes into spasm, the tensor veli palatini also can contract because of the spasm/contraction feedback mechanism. Hence, with closed eustachian tubes, and an inability to equalize middle-ear pressure, a patient can experience symptoms that mimic middle-ear problems.

Another frequently reported symptom is numbness in the hands and feet. There is a logical, if a bit complicated, reason for this. The spinal column encloses the spinal cord, which is the main nerve network connecting the brain to the rest of the body. Nerves move from inside the spinal column to the outside by passing through openings between the bones of the spinal column. Because of the interweaving of muscles between the bones of the spinal column, the nerves must pass between layers of muscles. If these muscles are in spasm, they may squeeze the nerves as they travel from the cord to the fingers or toes. This can create numbness, which can be mistaken for symptoms of neurological problems.

TMJ is basically a muscle-spasm problem. Because of this, standard diagnostic tests, blood work-ups, EEGs, or X-rays yield no information for a correct diagnosis. Often a sufferer is led to believe that little can be done for the problem except to block the pain rather than attacking the reason for it. Sometimes a label is put on the headache—migraine is a common one—not as a true diagnosis, but in an effort to calm the patient. In many cases, attempts to relieve the pain are in vain, leaving the TMJ patient suffering and often feeling helpless.

THE PROBLEM AND THE SYMPTOMS

Although some people with tooth-gearing problems have muscle spasms, others with the same problems don't. Why are some patients with a tooth-gearing problem symptomatic and others not? Why do people with symptoms experience them with such varying severity and frequency?

We don't know why some people are susceptible to muscle spasms; this is still a medical mystery. We can only observe that some people appear to be more susceptible than others. This is the same kind of mystery as why some people rarely have infections or colds, and others exposed to the same environment are constantly sick. Some people seem to be constitutionally stronger than others.

Susceptibility, pain, and the pain threshold concept can't be separated when discussing muscle spasms and their accompanying symptoms. When a person's threshold to pain is high, a muscle spasm may occur without pain. A person becomes symptomatic when either the spasm becomes worse or the patient's pain threshold drops. Sometimes both of these things happen.

It's still a mystery why a person's threshold to pain changes, although stress is sometimes given as a cause. We also don't know at what point a patient will experience pain with a muscle spasm. However, the degree of the muscle spasm will go up and down in the course of the day in response to varying stress levels. At a certain point, a spasm will be felt as pain. The threshold level is the point at which the person experiences pain.

We know that a person's threshold to stimuli tends to increase as the stimuli remain. If we cut ourselves, we may feel no pain at first and then experience intense pain when we begin tending to the cut. But, as we know from experiencing this kind of injury, the pain usually drops to a tolerable level after a short time.

With TMJ problems that become symptomatic, we don't know for sure if stress necessarily lowers the threshold or increases the spasm. Perhaps both of these things happen. But because the level of spasms and threshold change constantly, people sometimes have intermittent symptoms: bouts with neck and shoulder aches on stressful days, headaches at five in the afternoon every day, more severe symptoms when the body is stressed by unrelated illness, or headaches when especially tired.

When people have mild headaches, for example, and take an over-the-counter pain reliever, the central nervous system's response to the pain stimulus changes. In effect, when the pain reliever works, the person no longer feels the pain because his or her threshold has been raised. However, with TMJ patients, when symptoms are severe, neither over-the-counter medications nor prescription drugs are effective in raising the patient's threshold to the pain stimulus caused by the muscle spasms.

HELP AVAILABLE

Much can be done to correct the source of the muscle spasm and eliminate symptoms. But treating TMJ symptoms can't even begin until the problem is diagnosed. Treatment for TMJ depends on an accurate diagnosis of the condition. Fortunately, as described in the next chapter, diagnostic techniques are available.

3
Diagnosis of TMJ

It's not possible that my dizziness could be caused by my teeth! —a 60-year-old businessman

Coming here is my last hope. —a 40-year-old nurse

Diagnosis of TMJ is both simple and complex. This sounds paradoxical, but it isn't. The simple element is a screening process that can—and should—be a part of routine examinations of all dental patients. This simple screening procedure should also be a part of the diagnostic process for every patient who seeks medical help for headaches and other symptoms of TMJ.

THE VALUE OF SCREENING

Although the average dental patient is seldom experiencing TMJ symptoms, a positive finding in the screening can at times be crucial. Few people who have a positive screening for TMJ will need the more complex diagnostic procedures or treatment for the condition. These are usually reserved for patients who are symptomatic or need sophisticated dental procedures. But, in a small percentage of people, just knowing they have a propensity for TMJ problems can save many years of anguish and perhaps thousands of dollars in fruitless medical investigation and treatment should they become symptomatic. A positive TMJ screening simply informs the health care professional and the patient that the patient is a potential TMJ sufferer.

An example will illustrate the value of TMJ screening. Recently I received a call from Jim Murray, a former patient who'd had a positive screening for TMJ. He'd relocated to Ohio, and a few months before he decided to call me, he'd begun having regular headaches. "They started out mild, but now they're severe," he said. "I have a headache every day, and they're interfering with my life in a serious way. I can hardly make it through the day at work, let alone have a normal social life. I can trace the beginning of the headaches to a skiing accident I had. I was bruised and had a cracked rib that healed without difficulty, but shortly after the accident my headaches started. And I remembered what you told me the first time I saw you for a checkup."

I had told Mr. Murray the same thing I tell all my patients with a positive finding for TMJ:

You have a tooth-gearing problem. The vast majority of people do. Chances are you will never have symptoms of TMJ serious enough to be treated. But if you begin having regular headaches, neck or shoulder pain, backaches, popping or clicking in your jaw, numbness of the extremities, or middle-ear symptoms, then make sure TMJ is considered in the diagnostic investigation into your problem. In your case TMJ should be considered one of the primary possibilities, and keeping that in mind could save you enormous frustration, lengthy bouts with pain, and money spent in diagnostic procedures.

It's always heartening when a patient remembers this information. In the case of the injured skier, his memory of the TMJ screening gave him information about the possible cause of his pain. He was then able to seek an evaluation. The examination confirmed that the source of his pain was TMJ. We worked out an appropriate treatment plan, which ultimately relieved him of his problem.

Unfortunately, this kind of case is less common than the patients who see me after seeking help from numerous medical specialists. One patient with a positive TMJ screening had forgotten the advice she received. She looked for answers to her problem of severe headaches for a year before she remembered to consider an evaluation for TMJ. She'd been hospitalized, been given multiple batteries of tests, and even had two brain scans before she thought of TMJ. Once a TMJ evaluation uncovered the source of her pain, she was on the road back to a normal life. Within two months she was substantially pain-free; four months later her treatment was complete.

THE SCREENING PROCESS

It seems difficult to believe that a condition that causes so many problems can actually be detected in a matter of seconds. In an initial TMJ screening, patients are asked if they have experienced any of the common symptoms of the problem. Regardless of the outcome of the symptom check, the next step is examination of the external pterygoid muscles to see whether they are in spasm. This involves applying light pressure—a few ounces—to the muscle while observing the patient's responses. The response gives an indication of whether or not the muscle is in spasm. If it is, the touch is mildly to severely painful.

Sometimes a patient will show a response but deny feeling any pain. I often examine people who, while they appear not to respond, have an unmistakable look of pain in their eyes. As any person trained in the healing arts knows, the eyes give away pain. Sometimes people deny any symptoms, except for an occasional headache, or any discomfort when pressure is applied to the external pterygoids. My examination reveals that many of these people do have some indications of TMJ. But they answer the questions quickly, without thinking about them, because they sometimes think the questions are so out of the ordinary for a dental visit. They expect a question about head, neck, and shoulder pain about as much as they expect me to ask them about bunions.

Many patients havè spasms in the external pterygoid muscles but have no symptoms at all. These patients may remain that way for the rest of their lives. The TMJ screening only evaluates a predisposition to the problem.

Part of the screening procedure is a look at the motion of the jaw (its gait) to quickly evaluate the gearing of the teeth. In patients with tooth-gearing problems, the jaw usually makes a "detour" to the right or left as it opens and closes. The gait of the jaw gives preliminary information whether a tooth-gearing problem exists. Still, many patients have muscle spasms and a tooth-gearing problem but no symptoms of TMJ.

At this point, the actual screening—taking only a few minutes—is over. For the vast majority of patients, a positive response to the TMJ screening yields important information to be filed away in case it is ever needed. No further investigation into this problem is required. Mr. Murray's case was certainly a classic example of how useful the screening process is.

Remember that if a patient responds positively to a TMJ screening and later has symptoms similar to those of the condition, the positive screening does not necessarily mean that the symptoms are being caused by TMJ. The symptoms of TMJ are common to many physical and psychological disorders. Just as it's necessary for physicians to be aware of TMJ, it is also crucial that dentists not fall into the trap of believing that all headaches are caused by TMJ. However, it's been my experience that most symptomatic patients have had other causes of their pain ruled out before seeking TMJ evaluation.

FULL EVALUATION

At what point should a positive screen for TMJ be followed up with further diagnostic techniques and evaluation? The answer is twofold. If a patient seeks help *because* of symptoms, then a full diagnostic evaluation is done routinely. If the symptoms come to light in the course of an interview, then a complete diagnostic evaluation may also be appropriate. Many patients have symptoms that are so mild that they don't choose to follow up diagnosis with treatment. Others are in such intense pain that they are desperate for help.

There are other circumstances where diagnostic procedures are crucial. Sometimes a positive finding in the screening can extensively alter a standard dental treatment plan for a patient. The treatment plan may include treating TMJ as a primary and vital step even when the patient is not experiencing symptoms at the time. The best way to illustrate this is to cite some examples where further investigation was advantageous.

DENTAL WORK AND TMJ

Marianne Williams was referred by another dentist for extensive dental work. She needed bridges and numerous crowns. Her TMJ screening was positive; she had a tooth-gearing problem as well as some muscle spasms. Ms. Williams said she was not experiencing any of the symptoms she'd been asked about. However, there was a good chance that proceeding with the needed dental work could worsen the muscle-spasm problem and cause her to become symptomatic during or after the treatment.

Ms. Williams was advised to address and treat the TMJ condition first, and then proceed with the bridges and crowns. All too often, a patient's expensive crowns and bridges have had to be altered—in some cases destroyed and refabricated—because extensive dental work triggered TMJ problems.

For many people with potential TMJ problems, dental work can trigger TMJ symptoms because treatment requires a certain amount of manipulation of the jaw. Gearing surfaces of the teeth may also be changed. The patient may not adapt to and tolerate the change.

Does this happen 100 percent of the time? Not at all. But there is no way to predict who will become symptomatic and who will not. Many patients with the propensity for TMJ will go through a lifetime of dental treatment, including dentures in their later years, and never show symptoms of TMJ.

Ms. Williams wisely decided to address her TMJ condition first. Her health history contributed to her decision. In the diagnostic evaluation, she revealed that although she was not suffering TMJ symptoms at that time, she had experienced them in the past. When she learned the symptoms of TMJ, she remembered that five years previously she had been plagued by frequent and severe neck and shoulder pain. Upon reflection, she realized the pain had occurred over a six-month period when she was under unusual stress. The pain gradually lessened as the stress decreased. She had correctly attributed her pain to tension, but didn't know that she was predisposed to TMJ and that it was the root cause of her pain.

It's common for patients to look back into their own health histories and realize that they had, at another time, manifested TMJ symptoms. Had Ms. Williams known about TMJ, she could have addressed the problem, undergone treatment, and been spared six months of intense pain. Furthermore, had the bridgework been done prior to TMJ treatment, the problem might have been retriggered. At that point she would have had to undergo treatment for the TMJ and then a repetition of the dental work. Proceeding with extensive dental work without addressing the TMJ problems is too big a risk to take. Occasionally a patient will elect to do just that, but it is unadvisable.

PAIN AND TMJ

Sometimes patients go for routine dental care when, unlike Ms. Williams, they are manifesting TMJ symptoms. Some are in pain, but they have no idea their problem is related to their jaws. Often they get treated for the dental problems and no one ever discovers the TMJ. One case is a particularly dramatic illustration of how important this is.

Joy Rubin was not in pain when she gave her history. She had been referred for bridges in her lower jaw and expressed some surprise at my questions. Also, her neck movements were restricted; she was unable even to turn her head from side to side. In response to questions about this condition, Ms. Rubin revealed a number of things. Her stiff neck was a permanent condition; it never got better for even short periods of time. Every time she needed to look anywhere but straight ahead, she had to turn her whole body.

Ms. Rubin had been suffering with this condition for six years. It began with an automobile accident in which she suffered a whiplash injury. She had been to numerous medical specialists, including internationally known treatment institutions. She had also been under treatment with naprapaths and chiropractors but received no relief. She had been told to live with the condition, and for the previous two years she had become reconciled to living the rest of her life with restricted movements.

A thorough evaluation indicated TMJ. Ms. Rubin went home to think about the advice that she receive treatment before taking care of the bridgework. She needed some time to make up her mind because her previous treatments for this "locked neck" had falsely raised her hopes. When the various treatments didn't help, she became discouraged and depressed. Ultimately she gave up hope. It's often difficult for people to believe that a condition they've learned to live with can be alleviated. They don't want to face the painful possibility of being disappointed again. Of course, Ms. Rubin received no guarantees about TMJ treatment.

She decided to take what she called "one more chance" and see whether her condition could be reversed. She was taking more of a chance some twelve years ago than she would be taking today. The treatment protocol was neither as established nor as predictable years ago as it is now. Treatment began with the idea that relaxing her neck muscles could help the situation. The relaxation techniques were successful, much to Ms. Rubin's delight and relief.

During the diagnostic interview we talk about all the symptoms related to TMJ, past and present. The interview is usually quite lengthy. I want as much information as possible about the patient and the symptom pattern. When do the headaches, if that is the presenting symptom, occur? Where on the head are they located? How long do they last? How often does the patient have a headache? Other symptoms are evaluated in detail as well.

In Ms. Williams' case, her neck and shoulder pain history was taken in great detail. She had experienced a period of almost constant pain. Although her primary problem had occurred in the past, it could happen again at any time. I try to learn as much about the patient as I can in order to learn what might trigger the symptoms.

Because Ms. Williams had been under stress when her symptoms began, she tried to alleviate or manage the stress with exercise. She found, as do many patients with TMJ problems, that certain kinds of exercise make the problem worse. Bicycle riding had been one of Ms. William's favorite activities. Unfortunately, because of her tendency to clamp down on the teeth while bike riding, the muscle spasms became worse, and her neck and shoulders became unbearably sore. Even when the pain ended, she was afraid to get on a bike again for fear she would start the pain cycle over again.

EXPERIENCES WITH DIAGNOSIS

Mr. Murray had current daily headaches. Until he was examined and interviewed extensively, there was no way of being certain that his new headache problem was TMJ related. This was true even though he'd had a positive screening for TMJ some years before.

Mr. Murray's history was straightforward. His headaches had begun after an accident and seemingly overnight. The pain always started in his neck and moved up the back of his head and then to the top of his head and radiated to the temple region. We sometimes call this the "bathing cap" headache. His pattern was the same every day. He woke up with a headache and went to sleep with the pain. Sometimes he would waken in the night with a clenched jaw. He thought he was grinding his teeth as well.

In the examination, the slightest pressure of Mr. Murray's external pterygoid muscles made him almost jump out of his chair. Sometimes one part of the muscle is more sensitive upon examination than another part. The reactions, while unpleasant for the patient, help confirm that the symptoms are related to TMJ.

Mr. Murray came to the office in pain. Many patients do. Fortunately he decided to come in for a TMJ evaluation before he began to take narcotic pain relievers suggested by his physician. He was still coping as best he could with over-the-counter medications. Those patients who seek help for intense pain are often emotionally distraught as well. A few are almost incoherent because of the medication prescribed for them, and an interview is almost impossible to conduct. For many, their whole lives revolve around pain and attempting to cope with it. Sometimes the interview is emotionally as painful as the physical pain they are experiencing.

A woman named Julia Miller sought treatment in extreme physical and emotional pain. She was employed as a computer operator, her third such position in five years. A few months after starting the first computer job, she began having severe neck and shoulder pain. The pain became so intense that she became anxious every day about her ability to perform her job. Over a five-year period, Ms. Miller had lost two jobs because the pain interfered with her efficiency. When she finally landed a third job, she had been able to keep it only by investing a substantial amount of money in massage therapy two or three times a week.

Ms. Miller had reached a point in her life where the pain and anxiety had taken over her daily life—she was literally terrified of losing her job. She began to cry when she sat down for the interview and continued to cry after we were through. Although the muscles in her neck and shoulders were in painful spasm and she jumped whenever they were touched, the physical pain was nothing compared to the emotional pain she was feeling.

Ms. Miller, like most patients who have had the problem for any length of time, had sought help from many specialists. After she was unable to find relief, except temporarily from regular massage, she became depressed and also stopped talking about her pain to others. She lived alone, and her life revolved around trying to get through a day at work, and then relieving the almost unbearable symptoms through massage and other relaxation techniques. She also had a well-read library of self-help books on pain.

Over lunch one afternoon, a co-worker began talking about his headaches and how he had been "cured." The conversation occurred out of the blue, because Ms. Miller had never opened up to anyone on her job about her condition. In fact, she had come to believe that she was the only person who had ever suffered in this way. Her co-worker listened sympathetically when she finally decided to open up about her problem. This man remembered that neck and shoulder pain, while not his chief complaint, is one of the symptoms he'd been asked about. He convinced her to make an appointment for an evaluation. Because she had hidden her problem from so many people for long, going through the whole story of her pain was an intense emotional experience.

While Ms. Miller was a high school student, she had been treated for headaches that had been labeled as migraines. These headaches disappeared about the time she began working as a computer operator. Unfortunately, the shoulder and neck pain developed. While it could be that her earlier headaches were migraines, she may actually have had undiagnosed TMJ headaches. In her examination, even though she wasn't experiencing headaches, the various muscles in her head were in spasm, along with those in her neck and shoulders. Being a computer operator had forced her to sit in a chair for hours at a time, and her posture had been affected. Her symptoms had exhibited themselves in her neck and shoulders rather than her head.

A shift in location of symptoms is very common. The reasons for these traveling or "migrating," symptoms are quite logical considering the number of motions we put our bodies through every day. Our posture varies and changes as well. In certain people, putting stress on certain muscles makes them susceptible to spasm. The posture Ms. Miller assumed during working hours had shifted the spasm pattern down into her neck and shoulders. She may also have experienced mild headaches, but because the pain in her shoulders was so extreme, she didn't notice them.

A STORY WITH A MORAL

Of course, not every person in pain has TMJ. There are many many reasons for headaches, and detailed evaluation can sometimes rule out TMJ and lead the way to an accurate diagnosis.

One man whose most troublesome symptom was recurring intense headaches also had other symptoms that are classically related to TMJ—facial pain and numbness in the extremities and face. These symptoms had started some months after an automobile accident. However, the examination indicated that the signs did not go along with TMJ. The man had no tooth-gearing problem, and he was free of muscle spasms in his head and neck. The combination of symptoms suggested a neurological problem. He was referred to a neurologist and urged to look into his problem immediately. After a complete examination and testing, the neurologist diagnosed a brain tumor.

There is a moral to this story: It is important to be able to differentiate TMJ from other causes of headache and other symptoms that mimic TMJ. Just as TMJ patients in pain shouldn't miss out on appropriate treatment for their problem, neither should my colleagues in the dental profession and other healing arts treat all headache pain as if it were related to TMJ.

CHARTING YOUR SYMPTOMS

For many TMJ sufferers, symptoms seem to come and go inexplicably. When seeking a diagnosis, you will find it helpful to be able to answer questions accurately. What symptoms do you have? How often do you have them? How severe are they? It is also beneficial to have a general picture of the food you eat and activities you engage in throughout the day. This chart is one way of keeping track of symptoms. Possible symptoms include:

headache
earache
ear fullness
excessive tearing

shoulder ache
shoulder and neck stiffness
pain around the ears
mouth wetness or dryness

finger numbness
toe numbness
ringing in the ears
popping in jaws

pain in jaws
neck aches
eye dryness
dizziness

TIME	SYMPTOMS	SEVERITY (mild, moderate, severe)	FOOD CONSUMED	ACTIVITIES
Morning				
6:00–6:30				
6:30–7:00				
7:00–7:30				
7:30–8:00				
8:00–8:30				
8:30–9:00				
9:00–9:30				
9:30–10:00				
10:00–10:30				
10:30–11:00				
11:00–11:30				
11:30–12:00				

Afternoon
12:00–12:30
12:30–1:00
1:00–1:30
1:30–2:00
2:00–2:30
2:30–3:00
3:00–3:30
3:30–4:00
4:00–4:30
4:30–5:00

Evening
5:00–5:30
5:30–6:00
6:00–6:30
6:30–7:00
7:00–7:30
7:30–8:00
8:00–8:30
8:30–9:00
9:00–9:30
9:30–10:00
10:00–10:30
10:30–11:00
11:00–11:30
11:30–12:00

WHERE TO START

As TMJ becomes more widely known, patients occasionally see a dentist first, rather than seeking a physical examination. Marilyn Evans illustrates the shortcomings of this approach. Ms. Evans was a neighbor and long-time friend of one of my patients. Because they are friends, Ms. Evans had heard the "saga" of her neighbor's successful treatment for TMJ. When she began having headaches once or twice a week, she thought they could be TMJ-related as well. Her headaches were severe, and over-the-counter pain killers didn't help. She also tried some leftover narcotic pain killers she'd used after unrelated minor surgery. She made an appointment with me, eager to have her problem solved as her neighbor's had been.

Thorough examination showed that Ms. Evans had none of the diagnostic pointers to TMJ. When she described her headaches, they sounded like classic migraines—vision changes, nausea, a sense of flashing light. She was disappointed to hear the suggestion that she see a neurologist, who could help her with her specific problem.

EXAMINATION OF THE JOINT

A TMJ evaluation also includes an examination of the temporomandibular joint itself.

The joint is palpated; that is, touched or felt in such a way as to determine size, sensitivity, shape, motion, etc. We do this on the outside of the face in front of the ears, and through the ear canal while the patient opens and closes his or her mouth. There should be no popping or clicking. The patient indicates whether he or she is experiencing pain when opening and closing the mouth in this way. I always listen to the joint through a stethoscope as the mouth opens and closes; this gives an idea of the joint's overall health.

X-rays of the joint are another part of the evaluation. There's seldom anything unusual in the X-rays, but they can show dental problems, tumors, evidence of old injuries, and arthritis. A mass on an X-ray would signal a condition that needs attention from other specialists.

The jaw is also manipulated to determine the discrepancy between the way the teeth *do* gear and where they *would gear* if the existing teeth did not pull the jaw out of alignment. Fillings and other dental work are examined to see how they contribute to the problem.

A detailed interview and an oral examination are the core of the evaluation. The X-rays merely screen the patient for rare problems that may be contributing to the TMJ. The examination confirms, denies, or quantifies impressions formed during the interview process.

Headaches are the most common symptom produced as the result of the muscle spasms caused by the tooth-gearing problem; by no means are they the only one. You may have headaches and none of the other symptoms, or all of the others and no headaches at all. You may have one or three or five of the others without having connected them. It's important to examine all the common symptom groups found in people with TMJ problems, and explain and discuss how and why they occur in susceptible people.

4
An Overview of Headaches

The headache is one of the oldest human
diseases, and one of the most common. If you have any
doubt about the universality of headaches, a quick look at
television, radio, or magazine advertising should convince
you. Most of the ads for painkillers are targeted to the
headache sufferer. Headaches are often considered a normal
outcome of lives filled with daily stress and tension, an
unavoidable part of modern living. Americans spend close
to a billion dollars a year on over-the-counter pain relievers
to help them cope with this "normal" complaint.

A headache is unlike pain in any other part of the body.
If you have a pain in your arm, you may be disabled in
some way, but usually you can separate that pain from your
thought processes and emotions. However, pain in the head
attacks one's very emotional and intellectual center.

A CRIPPLING PROBLEM

Because headaches are common and seen as a normal part

of living, having a headache now and then is understood and acceptable. But only a headache sufferer who lives in chronic and intense pain can understand the way this pain can alter—even destroy—a whole life.

People who do not get headaches, or have only occasional mild ones, tend to suspect the sufferer is creating the pain for some psychological reason. This suspicion is strengthened by the absence of medical findings establishing a clear reason for the pain.

Having headaches is a kind of handicap or disability. Normal living is possible but more difficult. In fact, some very accomplished and famous people are said to have lived with chronic headaches. They evidently were able to rise above pain and live extraordinarily productive lives. George Bernard Shaw, Cervantes, Sigmund Freud, Lewis Carroll, Virginia Woolf, and Charles Darwin are only a few notables said to have suffered from regular severe headaches.

For many people, headaches come and go with no particular rhyme or reason, and variation in lifestyle has little effect. A headache can strike in the midst of a relaxing vacation or in the midst of conflict. Some victims of muscle-contraction, or tension, headaches say that relaxation seldom prevents the onset of a headache.

The language we use is rich in words that describe headache pain. People will say their heads are pounding, splitting, throbbing, or grinding. Or people say things like, "I feel like my head is breaking in two," or "There must be a red-hot poker in my head." Other people complain that they feel as if their brain is being squeezed in a vise, or that someone is driving nails into their head.

LONELY PAIN

Typically, a headache sufferer's pain has no direct connection to an obvious disorder or injury. Seeing an inflamed throat, a deep cut, or a sprained ankle, we expect that the person is in pain. But headache pain can be lonely and ultimately socially isolating. If the headaches are regular, the sufferers may end up hiding their pain in order to remain socially and professionally acceptable.

Patients have said that family members, friends, and co-workers have accused them of using their pain to manipulate others or gain sympathy for some hidden reason. One patient said, "A friend came right out and told me once that he thought my problem was in my head—but he didn't mean a headache. He thought I was nuts. I learned just to keep my mouth shut and not talk about my problem unless the pain got so bad I had to leave work or a party, or when I couldn't even answer the phone."

Some people—usually those who have little personal experience with headaches—think that this kind of pain is just an excuse. An individual who has a cold or a broken leg invites few questions by cancelling plans. But doubts arise when a person leaves work early, is in no mood to make love, or cancels a social arrangement because of a headache. Again, headache pain is lonely pain and open to suspicion.

CAUSES

Headaches may have one or numerous causes. A headache is usually felt as a single experience, but it could be a combination headache—one that has more than one cause. An evaluation of headaches must consider *all* possible causes and treatments. Not to do so is tragic, because today we know much about physiological reasons for the various headache types.

A headache can be a symptom of many minor or serious diseases and disorders. People often experience headaches with a common cold or flu, hypoglycemia, diabetes, anemia, allergy, and disorders of the eye. Other causes of headaches include tumor or concussion.

Anyone suffering from headache more than once in a while—especially if headaches are interfering with daily activities or increasing in severity or frequency—should seek help from a physician. This advice includes people seeking TMJ evaluation: Have a medical work-up for headaches first.

VASCULAR HEADACHES
The majority of headaches are categorized into two types, vascular and muscle-contraction. The most common type of vascular headache is a migraine. The term *migraine* is often applied to all headaches that are severe and debilitating but not life-threatening when no specific diagnosis can be made. In a way it's become a generic term for severe.

Migraines
More accurately, migraine headaches have their own characteristics and usually can be distinguished from other headaches. There are two kinds of migraine headaches, classic and common. In both types, the arteries in the head are painfully irritated and swollen. Both headache types generally affect only one side of the head at a time. The pain is caused by constriction of blood vessels, followed by their expansion and swelling. The expansion phase causes the intense pain.

Classic migraine is usually preceded by what has traditionally been called an aura. The aura is a change in visual perceptions—flashing lights, blind spots in the field of vision, confusion and/or lightheadedness, and often an increased sensitivity to noise. Some migraine sufferers report feeling partially paralyzed prior to the onset of the pain. A few say they also experience changes in their sense of smell.

Common migraine, also called a "sick" headache, got that name because it is often accompanied by nausea and vomiting. The headache is often preceded by a general feeling of depression or irritability. Some people report feeling a euphoria or an unexplained sense of extreme well-being prior to the onset, but this is rare. The common migraine makes up about 80 percent of all migraines; classic migraines account for the other 20 percent.

Many recognized medical authorities on headaches agree that some migraines are triggered by a substance known as tyramine. Many migraine sufferers can eliminate or reduce the frequency of attacks by avoiding foods containing tyramine, such as cheese, peanuts, chocolate, and red wine. (Many excellent books are available with complete lists of these foods and more detailed information about migraine headaches.)

Many other possible causes of migraine headaches have been identified. They include tobacco smoke, sun glare, strenuous exercise, erratic eating habits, excessive fatigue, and car exhaust. Migraines may strike weekly, monthly, yearly, or even less frequently. Some people report having migraines almost every day.

It is believed that more women than men are migraine sufferers. And, although it hasn't been conclusively shown, it's thought that migraines run in families.

Sinus Headaches

The sinus headache is a popular self-diagnosed headache. The pain is usually described as dull and aching, but generally not throbbing or pulsing. Sinus headaches are caused by inflammation of the mucous membranes or pressure in the sinuses, located on either side of the nose and in the forehead. Many headache authorities believe that sinus headaches are relatively uncommon. People sometimes label their headaches as sinus related because their pain is accompanied by a stuffy nose or tearing eyes. However, these same symptoms may or may not be related to other types of headaches.

Cluster Headaches

One of the most baffling kinds of vascular headaches is the cluster headache. It is thought to be a variant of the migraine. People who suffer from cluster headaches usually describe them as being truly unbearable. The pain experienced with cluster headaches is characterized by burning, searing, or a stabbing type of pain, usually on one side of the head and often centering around one eye. The sufferer may also have nasal stuffiness and sweating.

The term "cluster" is descriptive rather than diagnostic. A cluster headache occurs in groups. Each attack can last up to two hours, and four or more attacks may occur daily. Cluster headaches are said to occur more frequently during periods of rest, and this type of headache is more common among men than women.

Chemical and Environmental Headaches

Another group of headaches has received various labels and may be considered chemical or environmental in origin. The so-called "Chinese restaurant headache" is a good example of this. The culprit in this case is monosodium glutamate (MSG), a substance used to enhance flavor and commonly, but by no means exclusively, used in Chinese restaurants. If this is the only headache a person experiences, it is easy enough to eliminate it by simply avoiding MSG.

Some processed meats, such as hot dogs, lunch meats, ham, bacon, and sausage, use preservatives. But some people are extremely sensitive to them and get headaches every time they eat foods containing preservatives. This kind of headache can be prevented by avoiding the offending foods.

Other causes of headaches are also relatively easy to eliminate. However, identifying the habits, foods, or chemicals that could be responsible for the headaches can be difficult. For instance, exposure to certain chemicals will cause headaches in some people. Even a tiny gas leak in one's home can quickly bring on head pain. Eating ice cream too quickly has been blamed for certain kinds of headaches, as has eating too much salt. And headaches may occur when there is a drop in blood sugar. You do not have to be clinically hypoglycemic to experience a headache caused by low blood sugar. Skipping breakfast or lunch, eating too much sugar, or drinking copious amounts of coffee can trigger low-blood-sugar headaches.

Some people report headaches when they try to withdraw from caffeine. This kind of headache is so common that it now has its own name—logically, the caffeine-withdrawal headache. Those wishing to eliminate caffeine from their diets are generally advised to cut back slowly to avoid this kind of headache.

Some women experience a headache before the onset of menstruation. They may have one headache a month, and why this occurs is still a mystery. Many authorities link the headaches to water retention, common just before menstruation.

Brain Tumors

Almost all people who suffer from regular debilitating headaches will report fearing a brain tumor. Headaches caused by brain tumors are undoubtedly the most feared type, and these headaches share symptoms and characteristics of other types of headaches. Fortunately, brain tumors are extremely rare, and diagnostic tools are available to rule out a brain tumor early in the medical investigation of the pain.

MUSCLE-CONTRACTION HEADACHES

Most experts agree that muscle-contraction headaches are far more common than vascular headaches. They are the most common headache type of all, and for many people they represent an almost daily nagging of pain. Yet many people will call these headaches migraines because they are frequent and excruciating, and migraines sound like the most "serious" kind of headache. But much of this self-diagnosis and, unfortunately, medical misdiagnosis leads people to attempt treatment that trades debilitating pain for the use of drugs. Although great strides have been made in preventing migraine attacks and relieving the pain when one does strike, too many patients are told to learn to live with the pain, or dull it with drugs, or learn to avoid stress (an impossible task), when no reason can be found for headache pain and its related symptoms.

For some reason or combination of reasons, the muscle-contraction headache has been viewed as the type that the sufferers are expected to control by themselves. These headaches are dismissed, often cavalierly, as not particularly serious. Perhaps because they are so common, they aren't as mysterious or "glamorous" as migraines. Consequently, although muscle-contraction headaches are more common, much more research has centered around vascular headaches.

WHY ARE THESE HEADACHES COMMON?

In humans, the muscles of mastication are responsible for balancing the muscles in the front of the body with those in the back. This extra burden makes these muscles more susceptible to stress.

In addition, nature has provided protective mechanisms to ensure a species' survival. For example, many vital organs come in pairs, so that we can survive if something happens to one of them. For example, an animal can survive in the wild and we can survive in the modern world with one functioning kidney. We make accommodations in society to people without functioning ears or eyes. Yet an animal responsible for its own survival will probably not live long if it loses the functioning of both of its eyes or ears. Nature has also provided a strong protective mechanism for the jaw. Even if it isn't perfect, it will work and carry out needed functions, and the neuromuscular protective mechanisms will act to protect the teeth and their supporting structures. Unfortunately, this often leads to spasms in the muscles of mastication.

It may seem impossible that the vast majority of muscle-contraction headaches could result from a tooth-gearing problem. However, this is in part because of the terminology used for muscle-contraction headaches. This kind of headache is generally blamed on the catchall term "stress." But stress is often a misunderstood phenomenon. In modern society, we have been forced to adapt to increased noise levels, changes in diet, pollution, chemical agents in our food, complex family structures, pressure for achievement, and more. The list is endless. But it's important to remember that stress doesn't automatically make muscles go into spasm. A muscle spasm has to be triggered by something more.

Sleeping in a draft can make a back muscle go into spasm. A twisted ankle can cause a muscle in the upper calf to go into spasm because of the body's protective mechanisms. An injury in any part of the body can cause muscles to go into spasm. A tooth-gearing problem is one of the most common reasons for muscles in the head and neck to spasm. These spasms are the cause of the so-called tension or stress headaches.

PAIN FROM TOOTH-GEARING PROBLEMS

When we talk about muscle-contraction headaches, we're actually talking about a problem ultimately caused by a tooth-gearing problem overlaid with stress. When animals become stressed, they have an inborn reflex to gnash their teeth or clench their jaws. We can see this with dogs who react to strangers in the house. As an animal's stress increases, the clenching or gnashing increases.

Human beings have a similar response. We clench our jaws and sometimes gnash or grind our teeth in response to various stressors. Society also expects us to control or handle our stress, and in our valiant efforts to do so, we often produce more stress.

A tooth-gearing problem coupled with the additional balancing task of the muscles of mastication make the spasm cycle not only possible but extremely common. People who do not have tooth-gearing problems are not vulnerable to muscle-contraction headaches. However, because 80 to 90 percent of the population has less-than-perfect gearing, muscle-contraction, or TMJ, headaches are one of the most common health complaints known in human history.

TMJ and muscle-contraction headaches are actually synonymous. When people with gearing problems and symptoms are treated, their headaches go away. In TMJ treatment we see this day in and day out. The vast majority of people have symptoms of TMJ so mild that they will probably never need treatment. However, for people who suffer severe pain and other discomforts associated with TMJ, knowledge of this disorder will change attitudes and treatments within the health care community.

COMBINATION HEADACHES

Occasionally a patient describes headaches that sound as if they are TMJ-related. The patient then describes other headaches that sound like another type. Headaches occurring in one person are not always caused by one problem. Many patients' symptoms have a combination of causes. To a person in pain, it is difficult to differentiate between various kinds of headaches. People tend to attribute pain, especially if it is almost constant, to the same cause. As one patient put it, "pain is pain."

When TMJ treatment begins, a patient with more than one headache type can be confused about what is occurring. Within the first month a significant number of headaches go away. The patient is, of course, relieved; some even begin to believe that TMJ is the only reason for their pain. When the muscle spasms end and headaches are fewer, the other symptoms can be differentiated more clearly.

Some patients have migraine headaches that are "submerged" in the TMJ-related pain. Others have sinus conditions that cause headaches. Once the TMJ symptoms disappear, the other headaches can be evaluated. Often a dentist can help choose specialists to deal with the other sources of pain. Dealing with the TMJ component of the pain is a little like peeling away one layer of an onion. The second layer then becomes visible and can be evaluated. In some patients, TMJ headaches trigger migraines. Once the TMJ is treated, the frequency and severity of migraines are often drastically reduced.

WHIPLASH

Chronic whiplash symptoms, such as pain, stiffness, and restricted motion of the neck, have been found to be TMJ symptoms that were triggered by the accident causing the original whiplash injury.

OTHER SYMPTOMS

While headaches are the most common symptom of TMJ, this symptom seldom exists in isolation. Many patients report that they have few headaches but are plagued by other, less common TMJ symptoms. For those who suffer, these symptoms are equally troublesome and can lead to frustration and anguish. They too deserve attention in any discussion of TMJ.

5

Neck and Back Problems, Numb Fingers and Toes

My shoulders have ached for years and years. I thought it was normal. —a 45-year-old secretary

I'm numb one day and fine the next. There's no rhyme or reason. —a 22-year-old student

After headaches, the most common symptoms of TMJ are pain and stiffness in the neck and shoulders. They often occur with headaches, and patients report that pain begins near the temples, spreads to the front and back of the head, and down into the neck and shoulders. The pattern of pain resembles a knight's helmet; the entire head, from the forehead back, and the neck and shoulders are in pain. The pain can begin anywhere and spread throughout the area. The place the pain begins may be the same every time or change from headache to headache.

Backaches, both in the upper and lower back, are also frequently reported by patients subsequently diagnosed as having TMJ. When connected with TMJ problems, numbness in the extremities is a result of muscle spasms, not neurological abnormalities.

Like headaches, all of these symptoms may be caused by TMJ, by conditions unrelated to TMJ, or by a combination of conditions. TMJ may be one part, either major or minor, of an entire complement of symptoms and conditions. It is also important to remember that an evaluation of shoulder, neck, and back pain and muscle spasms should investigate *all* the causes of spasms.

Conditions like arthritis can cause neck pain, and anyone suffering with regular and persistent neck or back pain should have this condition investigated. Spasms in the neck muscles may also result from something as simple to remedy as sleeping in a draft. Occasionally people have to correct their posture in order to get rid of neck pain. People who walk with their heads thrust forward can sometimes correct neck pain simply by consciously training themselves to hold themselves more erect.

ONE PATIENT WITH NECK PAIN

Michael Maloney didn't seek treatment for his neck pain. He was referred by another dentist to have extensive reconstructive work done. However, from the way Mr. Maloney moved his body and head, it was obvious that he was in considerable pain. "I have to be careful not to jar my neck," he said. "It's been sore for weeks, and my doctor says I have another pinched nerve."

The routine screening revealed that his neck muscles and his external pterygoid muscles were in spasm. In addition, he had a severe tooth-gearing problem, adding to the evidence that TMJ should be considered. However, Mr. Maloney said that he rarely had headaches and that when they did occur, they were quite mild. He also said he didn't have any of the other common symptoms of TMJ.

Mr. Maloney came seeking a particular dental treatment, but was told that he had TMJ and that perhaps his neck pain was related. As with similar patients, it was important that the TMJ be addressed before his reconstructive work was started. It was likely that either the work would trigger other symptoms or the work would need to be altered or destroyed if Mr. Maloney later sought treatment for the TMJ.

As often happens, Mr. Maloney was skeptical about these

recommendations. He had never heard of TMJ, and he had been told and was accepting that his pain was caused by a pinched nerve. He decided to wait to have the dental work done, however, because he didn't want the additional discomfort while his neck still bothered him. He couldn't understand or believe that his pain could be connected with his teeth.

Mr. Maloney made his next appointment about a year later. He'd been through several more episodes of neck pain, and they were becoming more frequent and more severe. This time he was anxious to begin treatment for TMJ, partly because of his discomfort, but also because his physician had become more aware of TMJ and advised him to get help.

TREATING PAIN

This case demonstrates some important issues in the treatment of pain syndromes. Mr. Maloney's neck pain was diagnosed as a pinched nerve because, given the description of the symptoms, it was a logical explanation for the pain, and other reasons for the pain had been ruled out. This diagnosis was a descriptive diagnosis rather than an absolute one. Much pain experienced in the neck, shoulders, and back receives this kind of descriptive diagnosis rather than a definitive explanation.

A descriptive diagnosis has a number of ramifications for a patient. First, the patient is reassured that the condition isn't life-threatening. Second, it gives the patient a label for the pain—a name to put on a condition to explain it to friends, family, and co-workers. However, for a diagnosis based on a reasonable explanation of the pain, rather than the true cause, the only treatment is often pain-relief medication to help the patient cope through intense periods of discomfort.

When he first came to my office, Mr. Maloney managed to cope with the level of pain he was experiencing. But as the year went by, his threshold was lowered, he could no longer tolerate living with the periods of discomfort, and he eventually got fed up with the problem. He also had been given another possible reason for the symptom. He was then able to reevaluate his treatment choices. Once aware of TMJ, he began to be aware of how he clenched his teeth, and he could even feel the tooth-gearing discrepancy. Furthermore, he now had another health practitioner tell him that he might find help elsewhere.

As TMJ becomes more widely known within the health care community, more patients are likely to be referred for TMJ evaluation; they will get more than a descriptive diagnosis. This was advantageous for Mr. Maloney, because he was pain-free within two weeks of beginning treatment.

SORE SHOULDERS

Another manifestation of TMJ that usually is combined with other symptoms is shoulder pain and stiffness. Generally this symptom accompanies headaches and neck pain. We don't know why certain muscles become significantly more susceptible to painful spasms than others. However, we could speculate that posture places more physical stress on those muscles, depending upon the type of work a person does or the activities he or she engages in.

Mr. Maloney was a carpenter and spent much of the day leaning over, looking up, kneeling, and lifting. The muscles in his neck were the most susceptible to stress from these activites. Other people doing similar work may complain of shoulder pain and never mention neck discomfort. Many, if not most, people occasionally have sore shoulders. They usually attribute it to things like sitting at a desk too long, playing tennis too hard, or sleeping in an awkward position.

Shoulder pain is often caused by simple, everyday activities. In women, one common cause of shoulder pain is carrying a heavy bag over one shoulder. For many women this is a daily activity. However, some people with TMJ notice that after treament this stops being a significant problem.

Sore shoulders can result from injury to the shoulder joints, tendons, ligaments, or muscles. Muscle spasms themselves seldom damage the muscle. Arthritis and bursitis are also causes of shoulder and joint pain. Any person who has persistent pain of any kind should see a physician to have all these causes investigated.

Like headaches, shoulder pain can have more than one cause, resulting in confusion in diagnosis and treatment. This was the case with Margaret Adams. Ms. Adams had suffered with pain in one shoulder for many years. It was diagnosed as bursitis, and she had been under treatment for many years for that condition. She logically blamed all her shoulder pain on her diagnosed bursitis.

However, Ms. Adams also had frequent headaches and sought treatment for TMJ. She really didn't expect any resolution of her shoulder pain. During treatment, she noticed that her shoulder pain was less frequent and less severe. TMJ treatment eliminated one component of the shoulder problem, relieving much of her pain, and isolating her additional condition, thus making it easier to treat.

BACK PAIN

Back pain can have so many causes that entire books have been written about it. A person who complains of regular back pain should have all other possible causes investigated and eliminated before TMJ is considered. This is especially true if the person has no headaches or any other common symptoms of TMJ.

Back pain can be caused by structural problems in the spine and discs. Posture problems can produce back pain, with or without accompanying TMJ. An infection in the kidneys or in other internal organs can cause pain in the back, and even a peptic ulcer can cause this symptom.

Muscle spasms may also be caused by back strain from heavy lifting or sports injuries. Strain in the legs or shoulders may be felt as pain in the back because of an imbalance in the muscles in the whole chain. Even a slight injury may change the contraction patterns of the other muscles.

Any of these causes of back pain can exist independently or together with TMJ, and these causes should be investigated. When seeking a diagnosis, be mindful of the kind of diagnosis you are getting. Systemic diseases, herniated discs, and sports injuries that respond to treatment may not need further investigation. But when the cause of back pain is given as tension or stress, then TMJ should be investigated, bearing in mind that people with TMJ rarely experience back pain independently of other TMJ symptoms.

NUMB FINGERS AND TOES

Numbness in the fingers and toes is a symptom that alarms many patients. It is associated with neurological disorders, and patients often fear that they have suffered a stroke. Indeed, a physician should evaluate this symptom to rule out neurological disorders. A definitive diagnosis of TMJ shouldn't be made until all neurological causes have been ruled out. Remember, symptoms may have more than one cause.

When TMJ is the cause of extremity numbness, the symptom is related to muscle spasms. When a muscle is in spasm, it is contracting, and in the contraction it gets fatter. The increased "belly" of the muscle may press on the actual nerves as they exit from the spinal column and travel to the extremities.

Because muscle spasms come and go, numbness comes and goes. Variations in intensity appear to have less to do with the concept of dipping and rising of the threshold to pain. Numbness may occur with other painful symptoms or without it. It is one symptom that seems to have a time schedule and manifestation schedule that isn't predictably related to a patient's discomfort.

Occasionally a patient will report that his or her extremities become cold and may even change color, becoming very pale or even bluish. This is caused by the pinching of nerves of the tiny muscles around the blood vessels. Pinching or squeezing these nerves can change blood flow and affect the extremities. As with all the other symptoms of TMJ, coldness of the extremities and changes in skin color may be caused by other disorders. Raynaud's disease is a common cause of this symptom and should be investigated and ruled out before TMJ is considered.

As with headaches, while TMJ may cause the symptoms mentioned here, any manifestation of them should be considered a medical problem. If a physician rules out medical causes, the dental profession can be called in to investigate TMJ. Descriptive diagnoses—ones that only redescribe the symptoms without giving a logical reason for them—are not necessarily definitive and should be questioned.

6

Tooth Grinding and Facial Pain

Psychotherapy has helped me enormously, but I still grind away every night. —a 25-year-old dietician

I sometimes think the whole roomful of people can hear my jaw pop. —a 36-year-old actor

Grinding teeth and pain in the jaw, joint, teeth, and face often occur together. They may or may not occur with other TMJ symptoms such as headaches or neck stiffness. When the cause of these symptoms is unknown or incorrectly diagnosed, patients can be subjected to various treatments that seldom relieve the problems.

GRINDING TEETH

Bruxism is the medical name for grinding the teeth. Also, although few people associate it with bruxism, clenching the teeth is included in the medical definition. Clenching teeth is a natural response to stress in many animals, including humans. Bruxism can be directly related to TMJ, either as a trigger for the spasms or as a result of the discomfort.

Even though bruxism can be destructive to the teeth, it is not abnormal in all situations. In children it is not only natural for some tooth grinding to occur, it is desirable.

61

The teeth in a child's mouth often fit together poorly, and bruxing is necessary to refine the gearing parts of the teeth into a more normal scheme.

Typically, newly erupted front teeth have three bumps, called mamelons. In adults, the mamelons are rarely visible, because they have been worn off in the childhood grinding process. The only adults with mamelons have an "open bite," which means that the front teeth don't touch each other, and the wearing off of the mamelons doesn't take place.

Parents usually needn't worry if their children are grinding their teeth, even if the noise made by the bruxing keeps the entire household up at night. Any potential damage from the bruxing should show up in normal dental visits. As the child matures, the excessive bruxing usually disappears.

RESULTING PROBLEMS

Later in life, bruxing may become a way of getting rid of tension, anxiety, or nervousness. (It still can keep a household awake all night, while the sleeping person grinds away.) During waking hours, people relieve stress by clenching more than by grinding. A tooth-gearing problem may act as a trigger for the bruxing, which can result in muscle spasms in the external pterygoids and, therefore, may lead to painful symptoms.

In adults, bruxing can also damage the teeth and the supporting structures as well as produce painful symptoms. People with abnormal gearing of the teeth are unconsciously trying to grind away what doesn't fit well in their mouths. Unfortunately, the person rarely grinds in the primary area, that is, where the teeth conflict the most. Rather they shift to other areas and grind those teeth out of proper gearing. This happens because teeth that do not gear correctly are neurologically sensitive. This sensitivity may not produce pain, however. The body protects itself in ways the person is not conscious of. This protective mechanism will lead the person to grind elsewhere in the mouth.

A dentist can observe that some patients have ground their teeth just about everywhere except where the primary interference exists.

MOUTH GUARDS

Ellen Rogers was referred by a psychiatrist because of intermittent but severe headaches. She had also been grinding her teeth for so long that they were about half the height of normal teeth. She is by no means the only patient treated for TMJ whose teeth looked like tiny stubs as a result of bruxing. Ms. Rogers had a severe tooth-gearing problem and a full array of other symptoms, including neck pain, vertigo, and pain around her ears.

At her examination, she displayed a device she'd been using at night, similar to an athletic mouth guard. This device makes sense in that it keeps the teeth apart and prevents further damage to them. However, the mouth guard can hold the jaw in an unnatural and arbitrary position, which can then trigger further muscle spasms and TMJ symptoms.

Mouth guards are not recommended for TMJ treatment simply because the jaw isn't set in a natural position. Sometimes the patient gets lucky, and this arbitrary position may be proper for the jaw. In those few cases, symptoms will subside. But for far more patients, symptoms are exacerbated. Several patients have reported more severe morning headaches after using mouth guards than before using them.

TOOTHACHES

Ms. Rogers miraculously didn't have tooth pain along with the physical damage to the teeth, probably because the wear had taken place over a long period of time. Sometimes the mouth will wear itself into a position that the body can accommodate.

At other times, bruxism can go along with undiagnosable tooth pain, which is another symptom of TMJ. While this isn't always the case, people who are aware that they sometimes grind their teeth at night shouldn't be surprised if they have toothaches or jaw pain for which no apparent cause can be found.

There are numerous reasons for tooth pain, including decay, injury, a dying nerve in the tooth, an abscess, or a sinus infection. The reasons for tooth pain in a TMJ patient can be more complicated. Because a tooth has nerve material and tissue, it can become inflamed and swollen. Pain and sensitivity to cold are also early symptoms of a dying tooth. A dentist examining a patient will listen to the patient, X-ray the tooth, and tap the tooth with an instrument. Even though nothing is visible to indicate it, the symptoms point to a dying tooth. While other causes of pain are easily diagnosed by a dentist or a physician, in patients with toothaches caused by TMJ, the diagnostic process can be baffling.

TRAVELING PAIN

A patient once came to me for a routine checkup, and before I'd even had a chance to examine her, she told me that the previous year she'd had five root canals. When I questioned her further, she said that the root canal series had begun when one tooth caused her a great deal of pain. There was no decay or injury to the tooth, and it was eventually concluded that the tooth must be dying. A root canal was done; this was a logical, if not necessarily correct, diagnosis and treatment.

This treatment for a dying tooth wasn't unusual, except that a few weeks after the treatment was complete, she was back in the dentist's office complaining of pain in another tooth. The dentist repeated the same diagnostic sequence, and the patient had another root canal. This continued to happen until she'd had five of these procedures. Unfortunately, the pain still traveled from tooth to tooth.

Sometimes the pain will migrate around the mouth more quickly, and the patient tells the dentist that pain in one tooth went away in a few days, but came back someplace else—often, but not always, in the tooth directly above. Patients have been referred for psychological counseling because of migrating tooth pain. Since nothing appears to be physiologically wrong with each painful tooth, the cause seems to be psychological.

Most often migrating tooth pain is actually a result of the tooth-gearing problem. A cycle of hitting or banging the tooth is taking place. When a tooth is hit or banged over a period of time, the nerve in the tooth becomes inflamed. To protect that tooth, the jaw changes position to prevent the contact that caused the tooth to become inflamed and painful. Unfortunately, another tooth may then take the brunt of the hitting or banging, and it, like the first tooth, may become sensitive. The pattern can repeat itself indefinitely until many teeth have gone through a mysterious pain cycle. In many cases, this results in a mouth full of root canals. With older people, because the dental care available in their youth was less sophisticated than that available today, the painful teeth may have been removed instead.

"Hitting" or "banging" a tooth is a subtle process. No one consciously bangs a tooth. But in a patient who is grinding or clenching, the tooth may be taking the brunt of unnatural pressure, so the body unconsciously changes the clenching pattern.

REFERRED PAIN

The issue of tooth pain is further complicated because pain in a tooth can actually be "referred pain" from anywhere in the face or other areas of the body. Nerves send information along certain pathways. We don't know all the reasons for referred pain, but we know some directions pain might travel. For example, spasms in the external pterygoid muscles cause pain behind the eye. Similarly, pain in a tooth may be referred from some other place.

Problems having nothing to do with TMJ or dental status can cause referred tooth pain. Sinus problems, for example, may cause pain in the upper back teeth. The roots of the molars and the bicuspids sometimes intrude into the sinus cavities, separated by only a thin layer of bone and/or sinus membranes. Allergies may also cause tooth pain, often because environmental and food allergies cause inflammation in the sinuses.

Because we now know that mysterious or undiagnosed tooth pain can be caused by TMJ, this condition should be added to the list of possible causes for tooth pain. But because TMJ patients have the same dental problems as everyone else, problems such as decay, injury to the tooth, and abscess should be investigated thoroughly, too.

FACIAL PAIN

Facial pain is another symptom that can be quite mysterious and difficult to diagnose. Pain in the face is sometimes experienced along with a headache. People frequently say, "My head hurts so much that my face is in pain, too." Many people consider a pain in the head normal, but pain in the face spells alarm. Actually facial pain can be referred pain from a tooth problem, a sinus problem, or from an injury to the head.

There is also a condition called *tic douloureux*, which is a facial pain syndrome. It is characterized by intense short-lasting pain, and has a trigger point in the face. A person with this problem may not have any pain until this trigger point is touched. Patients with tic douloureux will actually shave or apply makeup around that trigger point. This is quite different from the facial pain associated with TMJ. Facial pain that is caused by TMJ problems usually lasts longer and does not have a particular point that triggers the pain. TMJ and tic douloureux can exist together. In these patients it seems that, as with migraines, TMJ triggers the problem to be more frequent and severe.

An occasional patient suffers only facial pain or perhaps one or two other TMJ symptoms. A few have facial pain with the cycle of bruxing and tooth pain, leading to a confirmation of a dying-tooth diagnosis. It isn't unusual for a patient to have facial pain when a tooth is abscessed.

PAIN AND NOISE IN THE JAW AND JOINT

Pain along the jaw should be distinguished from pain felt in the joint itself. Jaw pain is common when people have dental problems, and it sometimes accompanies bruxing. But it is also a symptom of a heart attack, and a person experiencing sudden jaw pain should not assume it is a dental concern or TMJ.

Pain felt in the joint itself can also have numerous causes. Sometimes the pain is accompanied by a popping or a clicking in the joint. This popping or clicking sound is rarely associated with pain. The source of the noise is the cartilage disc that protects the bones of the joint by preventing the bones from touching each other. When functioning normally, the disc is intact and moves smoothly and in a coordinated fashion with the jaw as it goes through its range of motion.

But if the cartilage disc becomes uncoordinated for any reason, it will slip out of position, producing a popping sound, and then making another popping sound as it moves back in. The disc can be out of its normally smooth coordination for many reasons—loose ligaments, lack of coordination in the muscles, a tear in the disc, or displacement.

Some patients never experience this symptom—it is common but by no means universal. Some people report this popping only when they open their mouths very wide, as in yawning or taking a bite of a large sandwich. The jaw also may lock at these times. The popping or clicking sound can be loud and bothersome. It should always be evaluated, because it can indicate damage to the joint or the cartilage disc.

These popping or clicking sounds are different from the sounds produced in other joint-derangement conditions such as arthritis. Joint derangement from arthritis makes a crackling, gritty sound, somewhat like sand in a gear. Often the patient can hear it, and the examining clinician can hear it with a stethoscope. In some cases, the sounds are loud enough to be heard by someone standing close to the patient.

This crackling or gritty sound indicates damage to the joint. This kind of damage can cause pain, and in keeping with the idea of referred pain, it's possible that damage to the joint may cause other symptoms such as headache.

However, in most TMJ patients, symptoms that seem to be related to the joint itself are not caused by the joint. They are actually caused by the muscle spasms most often seen in patients with joint popping or pain. The joint can't cause the muscle to go into spasm directly, and the ultimate cause is the tooth-gearing problem.

As will be discussed in Chapter 11, surgery is often considered the solution for people whose symptoms are directly connected to the joint itself. However, when muscle spasms are present, it is advisable to put off such drastic treatment until there is an attempt to relieve the pain with the standard treatment approach as it is most often successful.

Each of the symptoms described can occur alone or together with the more common symptoms—headaches, neck and shoulder pain and stiffness, etc. There are people with all of them and people seeking help with only one that manifests in a severe and debilitating way. Some symptoms appear to be related to the teeth and the jaw mechanism itself, but there are two other symptoms to be discussed which seem, on the surface, to have nothing whatever to do with a gearing problem in the teeth.

7

Middle-Ear Symptoms and Vertigo

I began to think I had allergies to everything.
—a 28-year-old writer

The headaches aren't as frightening as the dizziness.
—a 30-year-old artist

It's often difficult to understand how such symptoms as ringing or buzzing in the ears, earaches, altered hearing, or even vertigo (dizziness) can be connected to a muscle-spasm problem originating with the teeth. The connection is a small muscle called the tensor veli palatini.

A SMALL MUSCLE

The tensor veli palatini has a number of functions, including involvement in the closing of the eustachian tubes. This tube connects the throat to the middle ear and keeps the air pressure in the middle ear the same as that of the outside atmosphere. Normally this happens without our knowing it, but in certain cases, such as flying in an airplane, this change is noticeable.

The tensor veli palatini is supplied with nerve signals from a branch of the same nerve that supplies the external pterygoid muscle. When the external pterygoids are in spasm, the tensor veli palatini also can go into spasm because the nerve stimuli go to both muscles.

When this tiny muscle goes into spasm, it closes off the eustachian tube and produces symptoms that mimic middle-ear problems. A patient may see a physician about changes in hearing, earaches, buzzing, ringing, or dizziness. The patient may have no signs of infection or a cold, and when the problem is not resolved in a short time, allergies are often suspected.

ALLERGIES SUSPECTED

Mary Washington was a patient who'd been told numerous times that she had allergies because of the intermittent ear symptoms. It was assumed that milk was a culprit, because an allergy to milk will produce middle-ear symptoms in some patients. However, avoiding dairy products didn't make Ms. Washington's problem disappear.

Ms. Washington experienced dizziness along with the ringing and stuffiness in her ears. Dizziness has the same cause—the closing of the eustachian tube by the tensor veli palatini. Other patients have reported being put on antibiotics because of these middle-ear symptoms. The symptoms mimic infection and colds, and even when an infection isn't apparent, the symptoms are often treated with antibiotics. This group of symptoms is mysterious because the cause is almost never suspected to be TMJ.

This group of symptoms may exist with other TMJ symptoms or alone. A patient may have just buzzing or ringing and no dizziness or pain around the ear. Again, like the other symptoms, there is no way to predict which are going to occur and which will never appear.

Patients with middle-ear symptoms should realize that their problems could be caused by TMJ alone or along with other conditions such as allergy. Anyone experiencing these symptoms should look for other causes first. Ms. Washington had been on antibiotics before the allergies were suspected. It was when allergies were subsequently ruled out that TMJ could be considered. If a patient seeks TMJ evaluation and has a positive finding, it is likely that the middle-ear symptoms will be resolved during treatment. If a patient has TMJ and allergies, TMJ treatment will eliminate the component caused by that condition. The allergies or other ear problems can then be treated more effectively.

It turned out that Ms. Washington did in fact have allergies to a number of substances. However, until the TMJ was treated, there was no effective way to correlate her exposure to certain foods or environmental substances with her symptoms. She would avoid a particular food and be fine for a period of time. Then the middle-ear symptoms would return and confuse the determination of what she was allergic to. At one point she was experiencing these symptoms every day for weeks. She concluded that she was allergic to practically everything she was eating, wearing, and breathing.

DIZZINESS

Dizziness is sometimes blamed on stress. When no other cause can be found for various symptoms, stress is often blamed. One patient, Elizabeth Andersen, experienced dizziness many times a day. It came and went with no apparent cause. Ms. Andersen went through a series of tests, including an electroencephalogram (EEG), a CAT scan, and blood work, in order to determine the cause of these dizzy spells. Ultimately, stress was blamed.

Ms. Andersen tried to find ways to manage stress more effectively, but her dizzy spells continued to come and go mysteriously. More symptoms of TMJ began to appear— some neck stiffness, pain around her ears, and finally headaches. She sought help for the headaches without realizing that the dizziness could have the same ultimate cause. She was referred by a chiropractor who had become knowledgeable about TMJ. She mentioned the dizziness as separate from the other symptoms, but shortly after beginning treatment, that symptom began to disappear.

REFERRED PAIN

Pain in or around the ears can be referred pain from other places on the head or face. When the source of the pain is discovered to be TMJ and the condition is treated, the pain will disappear. But ear pain should never be ignored, and medical causes should be investigated.

When a person experiences dizziness, buzzing or ringing in the ears, or ear pain or stuffiness, and a diagnosis is made, a treatment plan should result. If the symptoms go away and don't recur immediately, then it is likely these symptoms are not connected to TMJ. But, as with other symptoms, many people are told that no cause can be found. They often are left with the impression that they must learn to live with the problems. People who have had this group of symptoms repeatedly investigated, receiving only tentative or descriptive diagnoses, should consider having an evaluation for TMJ.

8
Common Triggers for TMJ

I think it started about five years ago when I became a body builder. I never had a headache before that.
— a 26-year-old teacher and bodybuilder

I don't know when this began. I think my fingers and toes were always numb. I thought it was normal.
— a 45-year-old executive

The potential for TMJ problems exists in practically everyone—80 to 90 percent of the population has a tooth-gearing discrepancy. And day-to-day activities expose us to the common triggering of at least some TMJ symptoms. The absence of major symptoms in the vast majority of people is a tribute to our neuromuscular system's ability to protect us.

When a typical dental patient has a TMJ screening and is told that the potential for problems exists, this doesn't mean that the potential will ever be activated. The information simply lets the person know that if any of the mysterious symptoms of TMJ begin, the condition should be investigated.

TRAUMA AS A TRIGGER

Some of the triggers for TMJ are dramatic. A large number of patients seeking evaluation for TMJ can trace the onset of symptoms to some kind of trauma. Car accidents, sports injuries, a blow on the head or face, surgery, or loss of teeth can all trigger TMJ symptoms in susceptible people. Many other people suffer these traumas and do not become symptomatic. We don't know why some people will be pushed over the edge into symptom manifestation.

A common kind of trauma is automobile accidents. Even when an injury isn't terribly serious, a TMJ-susceptible person can become symptomatic. In a whiplash injury, the muscles in the neck are jarred and pulled suddenly, often causing severe stress. Sometimes the immobilizing collar that whiplash victims wear triggers symptoms. The collar pushes the lower jaw into the upper jaw and forces the lower jaw into a position that may be so unnatural that the external pterygoid muscles either go into spasm or increase their spasm.

Some people who seek a TMJ evaluation suffer an injury long before they actually seek help for their problems. At first the symptoms they experienced may have been minor, and it is assumed that they will eventually go away. For many fortunate people, they do, but for others, once the spasm cycle begins, it becomes established and doesn't go away on its own. For these people, the search for help begins when the discomfort seems to have no rhyme or reason and doesn't subside. They can trace their symptoms to some event, but they are told there is no apparent reason for the connection, especially if the injury sustained has healed normally.

Keep in mind that any kind of trauma can trigger TMJ. One patient could trace the beginning of his symptom cycle to a mugging. His attacker hit him in the face. He had no broken bones, but the blow was enough to cause symptoms, which included extremity numbness, neck and shoulder pain, intermittent middle-ear symptoms, and mild headaches. At first these symptoms were mild and infrequent, but gradually they became more severe.

Other people who have sustained trauma to the head and face will experience symptoms for a time, but gradually the symptoms disappear. The body can break this cycle of painful spasm on its own, and people forget these episodes ever occurred. The body's ability to heal is amazing, and more often than not, the TMJ symptoms triggered by trauma will eventually subside.

SPORTS INJURIES

Some sports, particularly sports that involve clenching the teeth, will trigger TMJ in susceptible people. This is a common occurrence among people who take up weight lifting. Any time a person picks up a heavy object, he or she clenches his or her teeth. This is a natural reponse to the stress of lifting. When people take up weight lifting, they may repeat this clenching activity many times in one exercise period. This is a perfect opportunity for the spasms to begin or increase.

Scuba divers also are susceptible to painful muscle spasms because of the biting down they must do on the breathing apparatus. This puts stress on the jaw and forces it into an arbitrary position that may trigger painful spasms. Patients who are divers often report experiencing headaches or other symptoms every time they dive. Many of them blame the headache on the pressure of being under-water, but it is likely that they are people susceptible to TMJ. If the headaches go away fairly quickly, people who really like the sport will consider it an acceptable price to pay for their hobby.

Any sport that involves either clenching the teeth or having the jaw in an unnatural position because of a mouth guard may trigger symptoms. Participation in various sports is fine, but people who are experiencing these symptoms should be aware of the possible triggers.

LOSS OF TEETH

Loss of teeth can trigger TMJ symptoms, although it may take years for this to happen. Whenever a tooth is lost, the teeth around it drift to fill the space. This changes the gearing scheme. Sometimes the body can accommodate the change, and no adverse affects are felt. Other times, a change, even a very subtle one in the gearing of the teeth, can trigger symptoms. Remember too, that even a minute gearing problem can cause severe symptoms. Yet some people walk around with severe gearing problems and no symptoms. We simply don't know why some people are especially susceptible to muscle spasms.

DENTISTRY AS A TRIGGER

Dentistry itself can trigger problems. Restorative work, as previously described, can trigger symptoms in patients who never experienced them before. A particularly sensitive patient can first experience TMJ symptoms during a period when much dental work is done. For some people, the stress of keeping the mouth opened wide is enough to make the muscles go into painful spasm. Numerous patients have reported this phenomenon. Something as minor as opening the mouth to bite into a large sandwich is enough to give some people a headache.

Patients will sometimes say that they knew, usually unconsciously, that certain activities put stress on their jaws. Sometimes they simply call it an "odd feeling" in the jaw when they have yawned widely, lifted weights, or started a jogging program. Some people let their mouths stay in a relaxed, slightly open position when they jog; others clench and even grind while they jog. If you wish to jog and you also experience even minor TMJ symptoms, try to stay in the more relaxed group rather than join the "clenchers."

STRESS AND TMJ

It is common to blame stress for many physical problems that involve muscle spasms, and patients often attribute their problems to too much tension or an inability to handle stress. However, this isn't a complete picture of how TMJ is triggered. It is important to remember that in order for stress to trigger muscle spasms in the external pterygoid muscles, a tooth-gearing problem must exist. TMJ is a tooth-gearing problem overlaid by stress. This nebulous concept of stress isn't a valid explanation for this muscle-spasm cycle.

Consider a patient who gave birth to one of her children before she had TMJ treatment. As any mother knows, it is natural for the teeth to clench during labor and delivery. When this patient gave birth the first time, she experienced severe TMJ symptoms that never really went away, although they did improve throughout the first year after the birth. She had TMJ treatment before having reconstructive work done, and her severe tooth-gearing problem was corrected. A year later she had another child, and she described the labor and delivery as much more difficult than the first. She clenched every bit as much as the first time, yet she had no TMJ symptoms whatsoever. Because she had no tooth-gearing problem, her body didn't have the trigger to start the spasm cycle.

Childbirth is a major trigger for women with untreated TMJ. If the spasm cycle becomes established and the woman begins to experience severe back or shoulder pain or headaches, then she is often told that it is the pressure of having a new baby that is causing her symptoms. While it is certainly true that the woman's stress level may be increased, her pain threshold may be lowered, or the spasms may have increased, it is the tooth-gearing problem that triggers the symptoms in the first place.

The physiological cause of TMJ needs to be emphasized when discussing triggers and stress, because many people end up placing too much of the blame for their own symptoms on some weakness in themselves. What they don't realize or take into consideration is that millions of people without gearing problems are experiencing stress too. These people might be every bit as tense as these self-blaming patients. However, those lucky enough to have proper gearing of the teeth aren't going to walk around with muscle-contraction headaches, and therefore they will avoid the stigma of having symptoms so long and so routinely blamed on tension and stress.

Most patients can't place any specific trigger on their TMJ symptoms. Many will say that the symptoms seemed to begin out of the blue. Others will link them with a difficult period in their lives; an equal number will say that the symptoms can occur during calm times as well as stressful ones.

After a pain syndrome is established, it doesn't matter very much what triggered it. What we do know is that undiagnosed pain can have tremendous ramifications in a person's life. One of the tragic outcomes of having undiagnosed TMJ is the way it can destroy a person's ability to live normally. As we'll see in the next chapter, TMJ can literally devastate its victims.

9

The Lives of TMJ Sufferers

Life? What life? I don't have one anymore.
                                    —a 46-year-old woman

*I don't live with pain, I live through it. And every day is an
ordeal.*   —a 31-year-old systems analyst

Anyone who has lived with, worked with, or
treated a person living in chronic or nearly chronic pain
knows that life can be extremely difficult. Many people
living in pain have only a semblance of a life. And as if the
pain itself were not bad enough, additional pressures and
concerns are thrust on people when the cause of the pain is
unknown. "To be in pain and be told nothing is 'wrong' is
one of the worst feelings I've ever experienced," said one
patient who had been living with excruciating headaches
and neck and shoulder pain for about six years.

During those six years, this patient, Ray Foreman, lost
almost everything in his life: his wife, his business, and a
series of jobs. His social life was a shambles, and he lived in
isolation and fear that he was really "crazy." Over the
period of months he was in treatment for TMJ, he related
many things about his previous existence. "My wife di-
vorced me because she thought I was using the pain to
avoid her, to avoid success in my business, and to control

people around me with the pain," he said. This is a variation on a common theme.

Finding a cause for pain, such as migraine, slipped disc, pinched nerve, or arthritis, enables a person to put a label on the pain. The sufferer can say, "I'm in this pain because I have a condition that is causing it. There's not much they can do for it, but at least I know that it's 'real.' " This knowledge lessens the strain on a relationship, career, or social life, although it certainly doesn't take away the pain.

PAIN WITHOUT REASON

However, many, if not most, of the TMJ sufferers I've treated over the years have been told that no cause can be found for the pain. The disastrous results of this message are manifested in numerous ways. Financial pressures often mount first, as the sufferer seeks help from one specialist after another. Meanwhile, the person may also be spending money on maintenance therapies, trying to keep the level of pain manageable. When one specialist after another can find no cause, family members, bosses, and friends sometimes become suspicious.

Mr. Foreman's wife started out sympathetic to his problem, and she supported his efforts to find help. Like anyone close to a person in pain, she was terribly concerned and feared that he might have some serious disease. She only began to doubt his pain when the months and years went by and no cause was found. During the time Mr. Foreman was seeking help, his symptoms became increasingly worse. His headaches began in the morning, then built to a crescendo of piercing pain in the afternoon. By evening, he was forced to go to bed, although he rarely slept more than an hour or two at a time.

During these episodes, he was unable to carry on any activity that is a part of a normal life. His formerly successful restaurant received less and less of his attention. Business began to fall off, but he was in such intense pain for such long periods of time that he no longer cared. He was told that the pain must be of psychological origin. He began seeing a therapist, but he couldn't begin to explore any possible emotional reasons for the pain because it was too severe for him to concentrate on the therapy.

It was at this time that his wife began to withdraw from him. "Our lives began to revolve totally around my pain. At first, she began to take days off from her job to go to the specialists with me, and a few times I was so bad off that she was afraid to leave me alone. But gradually things changed. She began to question me about the reality of my pain. Things went from bad to worse for me," he said.

What happened to Mr. Foreman is common in the lives of people with TMJ. After living a joyless life for several years, his wife confronted him and told him that unless he could find some help from a pain clinic or a therapist, she would leave. "We had no social life at all," he said. "I had to sell my business at a loss because I couldn't keep up with it. But even worse, our relationship deteriorated. She began to think the pain was just a way to keep from being with her. I had absolutely no sex drive at all, and she felt deprived of a normal life too. It was awful."

By the time Mr. Foreman came to me, he was living off his savings after trying to hold down a job and being unable to manage it. He was still trying to see a therapist— by now he was so depressed that therapy seemed like a logical alternative. It was his therapist who referred him for TMJ evaluation.

DEPRESSION AND TMJ

Not all patients with severe TMJ have lives as empty as Mr. Foreman's became, but many do. Long-term pain often causes severe depression, and unless a therapist is knowledgeable, the pain will be blamed on the depression, rather than the other way around. Often the patient who has lived with the problem for a long time begins to confuse cause and effect, too.

One patient was no longer sure about the cycle of

depression and pain. "There's been so much speculation about the cause of my pain that I'm no longer sure that the pain isn't caused by the depression," said Elizabeth Gomez. She was being treated for the depression with antidepressants, and for the pain with other drugs. It was no surprise that Ms. Gomez was confused about the cause and effect of her pain. The medication had severe side effects for her, including lethargy and memory loss. Although she managed to hold on to her job as a legal secretary, it was only because her best friend helped her out on the job, literally covering for her and correcting her mistakes. "I can't keep asking her to do this, and I'm not sure what's going to happen," she said. At one point she was considering checking herself into a psychiatric hospital. "I just wanted to escape and perhaps even be more drugged up. Oblivion sounded good to me."

Many patients are almost in oblivion by the time they seek help for TMJ. Even those who are managing to carry out normal functions often seem not to be "there" when being interviewed. Many people will fade in and out of periods of concentration and have enough of a handle on their lives to be aware of this mental cloud they live in. One patient gave custody of her two-year-old son to his father because she was afraid to be with the boy for long periods of time. "My ex-husband said that I was too out of it to take good care of him, and he's right," she said.

For some people, the effects of medication would be worth it if the pain were relieved. But for many people, the pain isn't gone. It may be slightly dulled, it may be less excruciating, but it is still there. Often the medication makes them care less about the pain: it will also dull them to the rest of life. One patient said, "The pain drove me crazy, but at least I could feel normal emotions. I don't cry these days, but I don't feel any joy either."

ACCUSING THE SUFFERERS

Sometimes patients are accused of controlling others with

their pain. One patient who was accused of this was Sandy Gilbert. Her husband carried a beeper with him at all times specifically because of her problem. When her headaches and dizziness came on suddenly, she would call her husband, and he would "rescue" her.

Almost all of Ms. Gilbert's friends and associates, and even her children, believed that she was trying to control her husband with her pain. They believed that these "attacks" were simply attention-getting ploys. The one person who didn't believe this was Mr. Gilbert, who not only believed the pain was very real, but almost never lost sympathy or patience with her problem. "My wife enjoyed life too much to deliberately ruin any of it with pain," he said.

Woman are often accused of using pain to avoid responsibility or sexual relationships. The "Not tonight dear, I have a headache" joke has become almost a part of accepted cultural humor. To people in pain who want to live their lives normally, it is a cruel joke indeed. Patients whose marriages have been disrupted or even ended as a direct result of their problems feel only despair at what has happened to them.

Many cases are less extreme, of course. Not all people with TMJ problems suffer chronic symptoms. Many patients will have severe bouts with painful symptoms for a few hours, a day, a week, or months at a time. Then the symptoms subside, sometimes for long periods, often for short stretches. Often these people have problems in their work, relationships, or day-to-day living.

Some people who suffer regular but not necessarily daily headaches are afraid to make plans because they are never sure they will be able to carry them out. "I've stopped making dates," said one young woman. "Canceling out once in a while is socially acceptable. But trying to find excuses to beg off over and over again eventually wears on people. Most of my friends think I'm at least a bit neurotic."

This label of neurotic is a common one put on people

who suffer from symptoms. People think TMJ sufferers are complainers or that they are weak; people may even accuse the headache sufferer of being a hypochondriac. Sometimes people who have TMJ seem to suffer from more minor illnesses and health complaints than people who don't have it. Pain can be exhausting, but it isn't unusual for TMJ patients to report having trouble sleeping. They may catch colds frequently or, in the case of women, may have more menstrual complaints.

Often after treatment, patients will report feeling better in every way—mentally, emotionally, and physically. Over and over, people say that they have fewer minor health complaints when they no longer live with chronic pain. Even though TMJ isn't life-threatening in and of itself, TMJ does affect overall health and well-being.

NORMAL PAIN?

Because headaches are such a common health complaint, they are viewed as normal. Many people feel that they just have a bit more severe case of this "normal" occurrence. Often these people live through the pain and by acts of will rise above it. They continue to lead normal lives, and in many cases "pretend" their way through it. One man said, "I never told anyone, not even my closest friends, that I had headaches almost every day. Not one person even saw me rub my temples, and I didn't tell people that I had regular massages because of the pain. They just thought I was indulging myself in a luxury item. It wasn't a luxury, it was a necessity."

Many patients are like this man. They don't complain, they don't talk about the pain, and somehow they manage to maintain professional and personal lives. Some homemakers even manage to take care of small children and run a household while in pain much of the time. These are the patients who seek help after reading about TMJ in popular magazines or hearing the subject discussed on radio or television shows. They identify with the symptoms, and only then do they tell others that they are like the people described in the articles or on the shows.

PAIN AND PERSONALITY

A few patients have talked about personality changes as a result of pain. They felt they were once pleasant people, able to enjoy others and have friends, but once the pain became more frequent and more severe, they became irritable and short-tempered. "My friends know when I'm having my symptoms," one woman said. "My sense of humor is gone, and my patience is almost nonexistent. I feel like a different and not very pleasant person."

Patients have reported changing their careers because the pain they were in made them unable to deal with people. "I couldn't sell anything to anybody when I was hurting. I became a proofreader instead of a salesperson so I could work in isolation. The pain was still there," a woman said, "but at least I didn't inflict my troubles on other people." This woman rarely talked to anyone about her symptoms because she thought they were just a part of normal life and no one could help her anyway.

People who suffer any TMJ symptoms over a long period often begin to view them as universal. Sometimes a patient will say, "Doesn't everyone have this popping sound in the jaws? I've had it for as long as I can remember." Other people begin to believe that ringing in the ears is normal. It becomes normal for them, because they have managed to ignore it and live with the symptoms.

TMJ symptoms strike many people. Almost everyone knows what a minor headache feels like, or shoulder and neck pains after a long, tense day. Most people experience these things once in a while. Minor symptoms can come and go and never have an impact. For these people, the vast majority, TMJ is insignificant and most likely needs no treatment. But, when pain begins to take over a person's life, all kinds of changes follow. It's tragic to see and hear so many stories of destroyed marriages and careers. It's tragic to know that many people are walking around in pain and believe that nothing can be done about it. However, treatment can help people whose pain is caused by TMJ. Most can become virtually pain-free, and most can put their lives back in order. Many patients refer to treatment as "getting my life back."

10

Treatment

I haven't had any pain in days. I can't believe it, but it works!
—a 42-year-old stockbroker

Now that I'm not in pain, I'm not sure how I coped before.
—a 28-year-old homemaker

Patients often think TMJ treatment is complicated and lengthy. They envision wearing mouthpieces, doing endless exercises, being hooked up to electrical devices, and attending relaxation classes forever. Some believe that surgery is probably inevitable. But when I describe TMJ treatment, as done in my office, patients are surprised at how simple it sounds.

I divide my TMJ treatment into two phases, with particular procedures unique to each phase. The goal of Phase I is first to break the cycle of muscle spasm, thereby relieving painful symptoms. We then go on to artificially achieve the proper relationship between the upper and lower jaw. In Phase I the lower jaw is allowed to move freely without the influence of the tooth-gearing problem. In Phase II we permanently or definitively correct the tooth-gearing problem. The goal of Phase II is to finish active treatment, and in most cases the patient is no longer a TMJ sufferer. Thus, TMJ treatment has a beginning and an end.

PHASE I

Phase I treatment artificially removes the underlying cause of muscle-spasm cycle, which is the trigger for the symptoms and signs previously mentioned. Remember that the *symptoms* are what the patients experience—pain, muscle stiffness, ringing in the ears, pain in the temporomandibular joint. The *signs* are those responses I observe or elicit from the patient, such as pain upon touching certain muscles.

Phase I treatment involves two basic kinds of procedures. Neither usually involves making any irreversible changes in the patient's teeth. Because the treatment of Phase I can be reversed, it can be used as a confirmation of diagnosis as the patient's signs and symptoms disappear. If a patient doesn't respond (this happens in a small percentage of cases), he or she usually hasn't been permanently altered in any way. In other words, a patient who doesn't respond is no worse off than when treatment was begun.

SPLINTS

A part of Phase I treatment involves placing a device in the patient's mouth. The device is commonly called a splint. Many patients I see, or readers of this book, might say, "Oh, yes, a splint. I had one of those, and it didn't help." Or some might say that it made their symptoms worse. Others might say that the splint helped for a period of time. Still others obtained full relief with the use of the splint.

Throughout the world, TMJ therapy uses numerous different kinds of splints and appliances. Some are what we call "placebo splints"; they have no therapeutic action other than to give the patient a sense that treatment is being administered. As with any placebo treatment, approximately 20 percent of the patients will experience some relief.

Other splints are designed to move or force the jaw into a prescribed position that is determined, sometimes arbitrarily, by the practitioner. Some practitioners believe that athletic mouth guards, custom or standard, can be worn at night and produce some results. However, the technique I have developed over the years and currently use is designed to free the jaw and allow natural repositioning to take place.

I developed my treatment splint after working with and studying numerous other appliances and devices. Although a small percentage of patients responded positively to the other devices, I became increasingly dissatisfied with what I considered to be an unacceptable proportion of patients successfully treated. Twenty to 40 percent is just fine if you are one of the successful two-fifths. However, that leaves many patients with little or no relief for all their efforts.

The splint is made out of plastic and is fabricated to fit inside the upper teeth. It looks like an orthodontic retainer without the wire going across the outside of the front teeth.

This splint is designed in such a way that when the patients put their teeth together, the lower front teeth touch the front part of the appliance and the back teeth are held slightly apart. This prevents the back teeth from gearing together and, in effect, keeps the teeth apart without conscious effort. This instantly eliminates the tooth-gearing problem.

The splint is necessary to remove the triggering mechanisms that program the neuromuscular system to keep the jaw in an abnormal position. Remember that without this abnormal "program" the jaw knows where it wants to go. The muscles, through the reflex mechanism, have programmed the jaw to go into a position that, on the surface, tends to protect the teeth, the jaw, and the temporomandibular joint. But in reality this protective position may send the muscles into spasm. The object of the splint is to allow the jaw to go back to its normal relaxed position. It doesn't do this all at once, but gradually in progressive stages.

With my treatment concept, only the front teeth contact the splint. This is done for two reasons. During treatment the jaw is repositioning itself. The splint itself creates an interference in this process, and the farther away the splint is from the joints the less effect the interference will have.

The other reason for this splint design involves the practicality of treatment time and the number of days between visits. No splint can be perfectly adjusted, and throughout Phase I treatment, the jaw is constantly moving in response to the splint. The back teeth aren't involved in the splint because the complexity of their gearing with the splint would make it almost impossible to adjust properly. If treatment progresses at all, it progresses more slowly.

So, we want the splint in an area of the mouth that is easy to work on, thereby improving the chances of getting the adjustment correct during each weekly visit.

TMJ is a problem twenty-four hours a day. The tooth-gearing problem that creates the spasms doesn't come and go. The muscles are generally in spasm all the time, although the patient's symptoms may come and go and vary in severity. When the patient wears the splint, the muscles start relaxing. When the splint is removed, the triggering mechanisms still exist. The muscles will then begin going back into their "limping" pattern. This, in effect, diminishes or eliminates the benefit derived from the splint.

For this reason, patients must be willing to wear the splint twenty-four hours a day during Phase I treatment. This is essential to the success of the treatment. The only time the splint is out of the mouth is when patients are eating or brushing their teeth. Some patients have said that in previous TMJ treatment they wore their splints only at night or for a certain number of hours each day. This is usually ineffective.

Wearing a splint erratically never allows the muscles to fully relax. This treatment might work for a patient who has mild, intermittent symptoms. In these cases the splint provides temporary relief—much like taking an aspirin. But this approach can't eliminate the tooth-gearing problem. Patients often say they notice the difference in the way their teeth fit together when the splint is out for the short, but necessary, periods to eat and brush. This is because of the muscular relaxation that has taken place.

Another question patients often ask is whether each splint used is the same. While the splints are basically all of the same design, they are made to treat each patient individually. Plaster casts of the patient's upper and lower teeth are made, and then these casts are used to fabricate the splint.

The device is seldom visible in the patient's mouth. However, because it is a foreign object in the mouth, it feels strange at first. The patient may speak with a noticeable lisp for the first few days. This lisp usually goes away in a short time, or it becomes so slight it's barely discernable by others.

An occasional patient may need TMJ treatment but for various reasons may be unable to have even a slight speech problem for a short time. I've treated actors, radio and TV personalities, and singers for whom a removable splint was unacceptable. In those rare cases I use a nonremovable splint fabricated on the patient's teeth.

The nonremovable splint has some important disadvantages, so I use this approach only when the standard splint is completely unacceptable. One big disadvantage is that it costs significantly more. Because it is fabricated on the teeth, certain dental procedures such as bonding or crowning must be done. This involves more "chair time" and office visits to get started. Any repairs on the splint must be done in the patient's mouth, again requiring more complex dental procedures.

The nonremovable splint may require initial definitive changes in the patient's mouth—crowns and bridges, for example. In the rare event TMJ treatment fails, the patient is left with both the pain and the changes made in the mouth's original status. This may require still more treatment in order to restore the patient's mouth to its original condition.

These risks and options are made clear to patients who require this kind of splint. Patients are told that treatment goals can be achieved with either kind of splint, but the nonremovable type is slightly more risky and much more costly.

MUSCLE RELAXATION

People who have TMJ symptoms are undergoing a muscle-spasm cycle—spasm, leading to contraction of the muscle, leading to more spasm—because of the neuromuscular system's protective mechanism. Therefore, it is necessary and vital to actively achieve relaxation of these muscles and break the spasm.

Relaxing muscles is not the primary objective of the splint. The object of the splint is to allow the muscles, once they have begun to relax, to function without tooth interferences. As the lower jaw moves toward its end relaxation point, the splint itself will trigger muscle spasms. That's why frequent office visits are necessary during Phase I treatment. We adjust the splint and break the muscle spasms during these visits.

Actively relaxing the muscles of mastication is just as important as wearing the splint. One part of treatment can't do its job without the other. There are many ways to relax these muscles. My technique is extremely simple in concept and application. However, other, more complicated methods such as drugs, electronic devices, and exercises have been used. These methods are outlined in detail in Chapter 14.

Over the years, I have found that the key muscles in the entire muscle-spasm chain are the external pterygoids. These are the only muscles responsible for directly opening the jaw. Most of the time, actively relaxing these muscles will cause other affected muscles in the chain to follow suit and relax without direct intervention.

Unfortunately, the external pterygoid muscles are not only small but hidden. Because of their location, they are impossible to massage. When they are in spasm, they also tend to be exquisitely tender to the touch. Their tenderness is a key to diagnosing TMJ in the first place. Relaxation of these muscles is rarely achieved by exercise.

It is well-known that when a muscle is in spasm, irritating it by some means tends to reduce the spasm. We don't know why this occurs, although there are many theories to explain it. As yet, these theories are conflicting, and we don't know the specific reason for this phenomenon.

You have probably observed this "irritation factor" yourself. When you have a cramp, or a charley horse, in your leg, you may automatically begin massaging it. At first the massage makes the pain more intense, but gradually the pain may subside and you may feel the muscle relax. You are achieving the same relaxation of the muscle spasm in your leg as is accomplished by breaking the spasm in the external pterygoid muscles in TMJ patients.

In the external pterygoids, the irritation factor is created with a muscle-injection technique. It is the most successful and comfortable technique I have found to relax the muscles. A tiny syringe is used, but unlike other injections, no medication is involved. The muscle is pricked with the needle, thus creating the irritation needed to relieve its spasm. There is little discomfort, because the injection is given in an area of the mouth in which there are few nerve fibers. And, as mentioned before, no fluid is injected into the muscle. The muscle-pricking technique is used in each office visit along with the adjustment of the splint.

In the vast majority of cases, the external pterygoids are the only muscles treated with the needle puncture. In rare instances, a muscle in the head or neck will be treated with this technique if the muscle is particularly resistant to relaxation.

There are many explanations for why this kind of technique works so well and so quickly. Some attribute it to the Chinese philosophy of acupuncture. Others base their theories on Western medicine's neurological explanation of why acupuncture works. However, no specific acupuncture points are pricked. The muscle is pricked wherever it can be

reached because the external pterygoid muscle is so difficult to get to.

The relaxation results from "irritating" the muscle, not
from stimulating any specific location of the muscle tissue.
In short, we don't know why this treatment works, but it is
effective. In my experience it is more effective than other
forms of muscle-relaxation therapy. The entire needle-
puncture treatment usually takes less than one second per
muscle.

I have also found that using a *very* mild muscle relaxant
will speed relief and the course of treatment by helping
break the muscle spasm. Using a muscle relaxant by itself is
not effective in relaxing the key muscle groups. Conversely,
not using it doesn't affect treatment results overall. In cases
involving pregnancy or a sensitivity to the drug, we simply
skip this part of the protocol. This only means that it may
take the patient somewhat longer to recover.

The drug used is orphenadrine citrate. Patients should
feel no side effects. In fact, I say, "The only time I want you
to be aware of this drug is when you remember to take it. If
you feel any side effects at all—drowsiness, change of
mental alertness, or anything unusual, then we know you
are taking too much, and we'll cut your dosage." Any drug
is potentially dangerous, and we use this drug only to work
on muscle relaxation. The dosage is minimal.

RESULTS IN PHASE I

The treatment combination of the active relaxation of the
external pterygoids and the use of the splint sometimes
brings almost immediate and dramatic relief. Occasionally
a patient will ask me what kind of drug is injected into the
muscle to create this relaxed, loose feeling in the jaw. Even
though patients have been told no drugs are used, they still
are often amazed at the swift response.

Most of the time, however, treatment progresses more
slowly. Patients typically begin feeling significant relief
within the first month—generally in the first couple of
weeks. Does this mean the symptoms will disappear one

day and never return? The course of improvement is, unfortunately, rarely that simple.

First, the severity and frequency of symptoms decline. Patients may notice they aren't bothered by such constant nagging pain. Some patients report that improvement begins when they no longer wake up with a headache. Others are more or less symptom-free for a few days, then for a day the symptoms come back with all their previous severity. There is no way to predict the course of relief. But, while treatment has peaks and valleys, the general trend is usually toward less severe symptoms or increasing amounts of time free of symptoms.

It's interesting to note that the severity and frequency of patient's symptoms at the beginning of treatment have little to do with rapidity of improvement. A patient with fairly mild symptoms may have a long, slow climb to relief. A patient with severe symptoms might improve rapidly. There is no way to predict this when beginning treatment.

For Phase I treatment to succeed, the patient must commit to weekly visits. The reason for this involves the constant and unpredictable shifting and changing of the lower jaw's position. On the day of the visit, the splint is adjusted after the needle-puncture treatment to relax the muscles.

Within hours after leaving the office, the patient's teeth are no longer gearing properly with the splint, but the muscles are seldom affected immediately. Toward the end of the week, as the next office visit approaches, the symptoms usually begin to return. As treatment progresses, the symptom-free periods become longer, and often the patient will be tempted to cancel the weekly appointment. However, early in treatment, this relief doesn't last, and the muscle spasms recur and may stop, or even reverse, the patient's progress.

Phase I treatment usually takes four to six months. There is no way to predict who will progress quickly and who will take longer to recover. But this portion of the treatment ends when three things happen in unison. First, the symptoms disappear. Next, the signs disappear. And finally, the movement of the jaw has stopped. These changes must occur together for a period of one to two months, while the patient is continuing routine weekly visits. Only then is the patient evaluated for Phase II treatment.

PHASE II

The splint has created an artificial environment in which the jaw can relax and assume a normal position. The needle puncture has relaxed and eliminated the muscle spasms. The result is a normally functioning jaw mechanism and relaxed muscles. The splint has allowed this to happen.

However, the splint, which has allowed the symptomatic recovery to take place, can have a detrimental effect on the teeth and gums. It's imperative that Phase II treatment involve the removal of the splint. But suppose we simply took the splint out and ended treatment. In the overwhelming majority of cases, the symptoms would return, usually in a very short time, if not immediately.

EQUILIBRATION

The options available for Phase II treatment depend on conditions in the patient's mouth at the time of evaluation. The most common procedure for Phase II is an equilibration. This procedure involves reshaping the teeth so they gear together in the way determined by Phase I. This is done using a dental drill to remove some surface area from the teeth and create a harmonious relationship between the teeth as the jaw goes through all its motions. With this harmony, further muscle spasms are unlikely to be triggered.

Equilibration usually takes about three to four hours and is generally done in one office visit, although occasionally follow-up visits are necesary. While spending three to four hours in a dental chair isn't fun, this procedure is usually painless. The amount of surface area removed from the teeth is minute, and the patient rarely needs to be anesthetized.

I am often asked whether TMJ can be caused by only one tooth being out of alignment. Although it is possible for a gearing problem to be exacerbated and symptoms triggered by a change in one tooth, this is rare. Equilibration is rarely as simple as reshaping one or two teeth. Equilibration is also often done on replacement teeth—crowns and bridges—or on fillings and inlays.

Treatment Variations

There are times when instead of taking away tooth surface, we need to add to it. Nowadays dentistry has techniques, such as bonding, with which to build up tooth surfaces. However, bonding material is not as strong as enamel and will eventually wear away. Therefore, when bonding is used to build up a tooth, it is a temporary solution used only to verify the success of Phase II. When bonding confirms that the teeth are gearing properly, the bonded tooth is replaced with a crown.

For some patients, an important part of Phase II treatment is to replace missing teeth. The loss of a tooth will not, in and of itself, necessarily cause TMJ. But when a tooth is missing, other teeth around it change their location in the mouth and often create an abnormal gearing scheme.

While treatment plans for Phase II vary enormously from patient to patient, the basic goal of treatment is the same: to make the upper and lower teeth mesh in a way that is compatible with all the motions of the temporomandibular joint. No muscle spasms are created, and there is no abnormal stress on the jaw. We eat, handle stress, exercise, and are usually blissfully unaware of our jaws and teeth.

APPEARANCE

A few patients wonder whether Phase II treatment will change the appearance of their teeth. Generally these are patients who will have equilibrations and perhaps some crowns. Some hope the dental work will improve the appearance of their teeth, while others are afraid the necessary work might flaw the appearance of their mouths in some way.

The gearing of teeth is independent from the way they appear. A person with a movie-star-perfect smile may have a serious tooth-gearing problem. The distribution of some other people's teeth is obviously abnormal. Occasionally a patient will tell friends who have abnormally appearing teeth that they *must* have TMJ. "You can tell just by looking at him," one patient said. While many of these people have the preexisting condition for TMJ, they may not be symptomatic.

Actually, few people have perfect gearing of the teeth. But in most cases the body is able to accommodate what it has to work with. It's when the body can't adjust to the incorrect gearing that the individual is vulnerable to muscle spasms and triggering of symptoms. And gearing problems and corrections might involve a "flaw" of one-thousandth of an inch! The eye can't see this kind of minute discrepancy. If tooth movement or reconstructive dentistry is necessary for Phase III, then significant changes to appearance are possible.

SOME EXAMPLES OF TREATMENT

What are Phase I and Phase II treatment like on a practical basis? The easiest way to understand the procedures and the way treatment progresses is to describe some specific cases.

A PATIENT WITH SEVERE SYMPTOMS

Remember Jim Murray? He'd been injured in an accident, and his symptoms started shortly afterward. His main complaint was headaches—excruciating daily headaches that seriously affected his life.

Phase I treatment with Mr. Murray proceeded at an average pace. That is, he began to notice a marked improve-

ment about three weeks into the treatment. I adjusted the
splint and gave him the needle-puncture treatment during
each visit. This combination often brought noticeable relaxation immediately.

During treatment, the external pterygoid muscles would
go back into spasm, and usually by the time of the next
office visit Mr. Murray was experiencing symptoms again.
But after about six weeks, he was no longer waking up with
headaches. Those he experienced, usually late in the afternoon, were manageable, because they were about half the
severity of his pretreatment headaches. About eight weeks
into treatment, Mr. Murray was progressing at a fairly
predictable and even pace.

However, one week he was unable to keep an appointment. By the time he saw me the next week, he was
discouraged because of the return of the morning headaches. They weren't severe, but neither could he ignore them
completely. He was also afraid the return of symptoms
could mean that treatment could fail. However, after the
next visit, Mr. Murray's symptoms improved, and his
morning headaches went away with normal treatment.

It was about three and a half months before Mr. Murray
happily announced that he'd had no headaches for a full
week. This indicated that he was probably nearing the end
of Phase I. We could then make a decision to go on to Phase
II, confident that his jaw had stopped moving. In Mr.
Murray's case, Phase II involved only an equilibration. His
total treatment time was about six months.

PREVENTING ONSET OF SYMPTOMS

Another patient mentioned previously, Marianne Williams,
was not experiencing symptoms when she came to me for
extensive reconstructive work. Because she had a positive
screening for TMJ and had, some years earlier, experienced
bouts with severe shoulder and neck pain and stiffness,
treatment was advised.

When a patient isn't symptomatic, Phase I is often very

short. We look for the signs—the muscle spasms—to sub-side. In Ms. William's case, this took about three weeks. Phase II reconstructive work was done to duplicate the pattern of the jaw and the teeth created in Phase I.

Ms. Williams's case was not particularly dramatic. She represents the kind of case in which we attempt to prevent the onset of TMJ symptoms. People with positive screening are advised to have treatment when extensive dental work needs to be done. In a way, it is an insurance policy that the investment in the reconstructive dentistry will not need to be destroyed at a later date in the event TMJ is triggered.

PROFOUND CHANGE

Joy Rubin's case represents a much more dramatic example of treatment that profoundly changes a person's life. Ms. Rubin came to me for bridges in her lower jaw. Initially, she didn't mention her inability to move her head from side to side. However, I noticed this in the evaluation and questioned her about it. She had lived this way for many years and had given up believing her condition could be helped.

At the time of Ms. Rubin's treatment, my treatment methods were still being developed. Had she undergone treatment five years later, the methods would have been much more established and predictable. Ms. Rubin knew a number of methods would be attempted in the course of her treatment.

Ms. Rubin agreed to come in for an entire afternoon of trying the needle-puncture technique on various muscle groups. I worked with the muscles, methodically eliminating the spasms one by one. The motion in her neck began to return. After the external pterygoid muscles thoroughly relaxed, she regained total ability to rotate her neck normally.

Ms. Rubin's treatment represented a breakthrough in understanding that the key muscles involved in the muscle-spasm cycle were the external pterygoids. This work with Ms. Rubin led to a predictable protocol for Phase I treatment. Ms. Rubin also wore a splint and continued to come in for weekly adjustments and needle puncture. In about four months, we were able to move to Phase II, which involved fabricating bridges.

This patient illustrates how TMJ treatment can significantly change someone's life. Although Ms. Rubin wasn't in pain, the restrictions on her range of motion seriously affected her life. Before treatment, she had been unable to look behind her without moving her whole body—potentially dangerous when driving and prohibitive of participation in any sport. Once TMJ treatment was complete, all the normal activities of life were open to her again. Once, when she turned around to talk to her young son in the back seat of her car, he said, "You've never looked at me when we were in the car before."

RELIEF FROM EXCRUCIATING PAIN
Julia Miller had also lost her ability to live a normal life. Her situation was worse than Ms. Rubin's in that she was experiencing excruciating pain. Her progress in Phase I was slow, with many peaks and valleys. She didn't begin responding until about three weeks after beginning treatment.

Throughout treatment, Ms. Rubin's symptoms would increase or decrease in intensity as her stress levels went up and down. However, over a period of about six months, the number of symptom-free days increased, and her pain became less and less severe. When she had remained virtually symptom-free for about two months, we did an equilibration, and she has not experienced symptoms since.

Sarah Johnson also had debilitating headaches. She had all but discontinued a social life, she was depressed, and the drugs she was taking left her unable to care about much of anything in life. Ms. Johnson's case illustrates that the severity of symptoms often has little to do with the rapidity of relief.

Ms. Johnson was fitted with her splint, and the needle-puncture technique proved dramatically effective. After the needle injections on the first treatment visit, she felt her jaw relax and her headache subside. She then asked what type of drug was used in the injection. It was nearly impossible for her to believe that her longstanding symptoms could be relieved with a technique that appeared so simple and involved no drugs.

Within six weeks of beginning treatment, Ms. Johnson was symptom-free. She also stopped taking pain relievers and spoke to a physician I referred her to about possible withdrawal difficulties. Regaining her ability to think and feel like a normal person, and living without daily pain, made her able to resume relationships with her family and friends, and even go back to work.

Treatment for depression and psychological problems seemed absurd to her once her TMJ was successfully treated. The only negative feeling she expressed about her ordeal was a completely natural anger at having had to go through so much before her problem was recognized. Her Phase II treatment involved an equilibration and restorative work—some crowns and bridges.

VARIATIONS IN PROGRESS

Barry Stern spent several months in Phase I treatment but needed only one equilibration visit in Phase II. It was a great relief to him to stop worrying about stress constantly. Once he accepted that his problem was physiologically based, he became much more confident and relaxed. He continued to run regularly throughout treatment, and learned to consciously keep his teeth apart instead of clenching down on them.

Sometimes a patient's progress is slow because of the type of work he or she must continue to do throughout treatment. Michael Maloney, the patient whose only complaint was severe neck pain, progressed slowly at first because his carpentry job required him to stress his neck daily. However, once his symptoms were resolved completely, after about three months in Phase I, they never came back. Phase

II took several months because he needed to have some orthodontics.

TREATING TMJ AND ANOTHER CONDITION

Occasionally a patient needs TMJ treatment at the same time he or she is being treated for another condition. Steve Smith was such a patient. He had been injured and had to undergo cervical (neck) traction. Unfortunately, he had undiagnosed TMJ problems, and the device necessary for the traction triggered symptoms. This necessary device transmits its force to the skull through the teeth. Another part of the traction device transmits the force directly to the back of the head. With a TMJ problem, forcing the lower jaw into the upper jaw may trigger muscle spasms. In Mr. Smith's case, the muscle spasms triggered severe symptoms, and he was referred to me for an evaluation when the pain made him unable to continue this type of therapy.

His treatment used a special kind of appliance that directly transmitted the force of traction from his lower jaw through his teeth to his upper jaw without triggering muscle spasms. He was then able to continue with the cervical traction he needed and later undergo successful TMJ treatment.

For patients having more than one kind of headache, the treatment plan requires sorting out the various types of headaches they are experiencing. Anna Martin, a beauty salon owner, came to me because of severe daily headaches, which she called migraines. About once a week she had the typical visual changes associated with classic migraine. Ms. Martin seemed to be a combination patient, because she did exhibit some migraine symptoms. However, there was a large TMJ component as well.

Her TMJ was treated, and by the end of Phase I the majority of her headaches were gone. She still experienced a moderate migraine about once a month, far less often than the migraines had been occurring. For some un-known reason, a TMJ headache can often trigger other kinds of headaches. Once the TMJ is treated, the other types of headaches become less frequent or even disappear.

COMPLEX PHASE II TREATMENT

In some cases, fortunately rare, Phase II treatment involves a complicated combination of therapies. Harold Barry received such treatment. Actually, his treatment had started long before he came to see me. He had suffered a broken jaw, which had presumably healed normally. However, from that point on, he had constant headaches and neck stiffness. He went from physician to oral surgeon to chiropractor and back again through the cycle. By the time I saw him, he'd had two surgeries on his jaw, but he still had the headaches. He also had undergone orthodontic treatment, but he was still symptomatic.

Mr. Barry was in pain when he came to see me, and his external pterygoid muscles were in spasm. Despite his other treatments, he also had an extreme tooth-gearing problem. Once the splint was in his mouth and his muscles relaxed with the needle puncture, his symptoms went away almost immediately. Mr. Barry agreed to continue with Phase II. Unfortunately, this involved still another surgery to reposition his jaw—a rare, but sometimes unavoidable, therapy. He also needed more orthodontic work to get his teeth closer to proper gearing. When that phase of treatment was complete, some necessary reconstructive work was done. His treatment was completed with an equilibration. Mr. Barry has been symptom-free for many years. Fortunately, this kind of complicated case is the exception rather than the rule.

THE PROSPECTS FOR SUCCESS

Once TMJ is diagnosed and Phase I treatment begins, the chances for success are great. This is in part because other causes for the pain generally have been ruled out, and the diagnostic evaluation has shown clear signs that TMJ does exist in the patient. This makes treatment failure particularly frustrating. A tiny percentage of patients fail to respond to any muscle-relaxation techniques, and their symptoms don't subside. We try for about a month to see if there is any resolution of the problem, but after that, the likelihood of success is very slim.

Other patients will respond to the Phase I therapy in terms of the signs. The muscles will be relaxed, and the jaw begins to move into a normal position, yet the patient still experiences symptoms. We don't know why this happens. It's disappointing, sometimes devastating, and can't be predicted before treatment begins. In cases like these, patients are referred to other specialists for further evaluation. There is nothing more to do for TMJ problems.

Most patients are able to complete Phase I treatment in four to six months. If they aren't symptomatic when they begin treatment, Phase I can be much shorter. Phase II is individualized, so time estimates vary much more. Some patients need a one-visit equilibration, and for others, Phase II treatment lasts more than a year. However, in all cases the goal is to treat the underlying cause of symptoms and try to ensure they will never return.

Most patients who have heard about TMJ or who know other people who have had various treatments for the problem have heard surgery discussed as a possible solution to their problems. In the majority of cases, surgery is not and probably never will be needed. But, because they are so often discussed and sometimes feared, surgical options for TMJ are examined in the next chapter.

11

Surgery

If I can't avoid it, I'll go through it, but I don't want to.
　　　　　　　　　　　　　　　　—a 59-year-old lawyer

Will the second surgery be worth the risk? It worries me.
　　　　　　　　　　　　　　　　—a 23-year-old student

At one time surgery was a treatment of choice, or the first treatment considered, for people who had clear, detectable, and demonstrable joint damage. However, surgery is seldom advisable until more conservative treatment has been attempted without appreciable or satisfactory success.

WEIGHING THE ADVANTAGES

In most cases, Phase I treatment will bring significant relief to the patient. The patient can cope with any symptoms that remain. In other words, Phase I may not relieve all symptoms entirely in a patient who has some joint derangement, but many people would rather live with occasional discomfort than risk surgery. This is a subjective judgment, and only the patient can decide when standard treatment has brought enough relief.

Susan Morgan had been told that she had a perforated cartilage disc, and corrective surgery had been recommended. She had some popping and clicking in the joint, but her headaches were more bothersome to her. Examination showed that her muscles were in spasm. It was suggested that she could try a less invasive method of treatment and if that was successful go on to Phase II to correct her tooth-gearing problem. If Phase I was unsuccessful, the surgical option was still open to her. A very large percentage of such surgeries can be avoided.

Phase I treatment relieved almost all of Ms. Morgan's discomfort. However, because she did have a perforated disc, she continued to have the popping and some pain around the joint. The pain was intermittent and too slight to make her choose surgery. She also was aware that if the perforated disc gave her problems later, she could make another decision about surgery. This was about five years ago, and so far Ms. Morgan has no symptoms that she considers important enough to warrant surgery.

The important consideration about surgery is that once it's done, it can't be taken back. And surgery on the temporomandibular joint is major surgery with all the associated risks. The single biggest risk of any major surgery is general anesthesia, and this risk shouldn't be taken lightly.

WHAT'S INVOLVED

TMJ surgery involves separating the two parts of the jaw joint. Plastic surgery techniques are used to prevent disfigurement and scarring from the incision. Generally the incision is made in the fold of skin just in front of the ear.

When a disc is repaired, the joint is dislocated and the disc is examined and sewn back together. Sometimes the disc is replaced with a synthetic material. The surgery also involves a hospital stay, varying from patient to patient, but often a week to ten days. During the recovery period, the patient experiences swelling and discomfort while the tissues heal. Total recovery time can be several months.

If this surgery were shown to consistently correct the symptoms of TMJ in the majority of cases, it might be worth it. But while these surgeries are most often done with a high level of skill and care, many patients end up disappointed because the problems may remain after the healing period is over. For this reason, surgery should be considered as an absolute last resort in treating the symptoms of TMJ. When the pain is caused by a torn disc or a problem in the joint, surgery can completely resolve the patient's pain. Thus, while a last resort, TMJ surgery is not unsuccessful in all cases.

A SECOND TRY

Sometimes a second surgery is suggested because the first surgery didn't resolve the patient's problems. However, sometimes patients do not want to risk second surgical attempts. This is often because they were made worse in the first operation. Linda James was such a patient. She was referred for an evaluation before a second surgery was scheduled. The first surgery was done because of pain around the joint. No joint derangement showed up on X-rays.

Ms. James was considering a second surgery because the first one made her unable to open her mouth any wider than a centimeter. The normal opening distance is three or four centimeters (about an inch and a half). She was unable to eat, talk, or laugh normally. But her distress came from the worsening of her pain.

There had been no way to predict that surgery would make this patient worse off. The surgery itself was done well, and Ms. James's problems may have been a result of the healing process. Whenever body tissues are cut into, scar tissue can develop. It's possible that her inability to open her mouth was a result of scar tissue rendering the muscles inelastic—unable to stretch enough to open the mouth to a normal width. Examination showed Ms. James's external pterygoid muscles were in spasm. It was recommended that she try TMJ treatment before the second surgery.

Because of the limited range of movement of Ms. James's mouth, treating her involved fabricating a customized impression tray just to take the impression on which the splint was made. Her jaw movement was so limited that it was difficult to get access to the external pterygoid muscles to give her the needle-puncture treatment. However, over a period of months, the pain gradually subsided, and she was able to open her mouth another centimeter wider.

When treatment of the muscles had gone as far as possible, Ms. James had to decide about surgery. Because her pain was gone, she decided against risking another surgery. She had learned to accommodate herself to the inability to open her mouth normally. She was afraid to risk losing that gain. Whether the surgery would have been successful is an unknown; it might have resolved her problem. In these cases, the patients must decide what risks are worth taking.

MAKING THE DECISION

In general, TMJ surgery is least justified when there are muscle spasms. A damaged disc does not necessarily justify surgery, especially when muscle spasms are present. Arthritis doesn't automatically justify surgery either, especially because the pain is probably coming from the muscle spasms and not from the arthritic condition.

One patient had two surgeries to correct derangement of the joint caused by arthritis. In this kind of surgery, the bone is contoured, and the disc is repaired if needed. In this patient's case, the surgery eliminated the crackling sounds. Unfortunately, the patient's pain remained, and he still needed muscular treatment and permanent correction of the gearing problems.

Patients usually decide about surgery based on the amount of discomfort they have lived with before muscular treatment and the percentage of discomfort remaining afterward. For many people, being rid of 70 to 80 percent of the pain is satisfactory, and they choose not to risk surgery.

The dilemma for patients is knowing whether they are among the small percentage of patients who will benefit from surgery. Again, this comes down to an evaluation of muscle spasms. In Gary Hynes's case, surgery was a logical choice. He was quite sure he had TMJ and came for an evaluation. His main complaints were clicking and popping in the joint and joint pain. The popping sounds could be heard with a stethoscope. However, he had no other signs or symptoms of TMJ. He was evaluated three times when he had the pain, just to be sure that no spasms or other signs of TMJ were present.

In such cases, the only logical treatment choice is surgery. Of course Mr. Hynes could decide simply to cope with the pain. But this case illustrates that not all people complaining of symptoms in the joint itself have pain caused by muscle spasms.

Any person who is advised to have nonemergency surgery should get a second opinion. This includes people who have pain in or around the temporomandibular joint. If the problem is caused by muscle spasms, the patient should try nonsurgical treatment, as described in Chapter 10. Only when that possibility has been eliminated should surgery be considered.

12

Treatment Costs and Insurance Coverage

The dollar cost can't make my life any worse than it is now.
—a 35-year-old public relations director

They say they will cover it if I'm hospitalized!
—a 29-year-old pregnant woman

It's difficult to talk about treatment costs for TMJ, because they vary so much from patient to patient. The costs are determined by the amount of time spent in Phase I treatment and the kind of procedures used in Phase II. Phase I treatment is basically the same for everyone, yet some patients are pain-free in a matter of weeks, while other patients are in Phase I treatment for many months.

Let's consider a general range of costs for an average patient. If a patient is in Phase I treatment for four months and has an equilibration as the Phase II definitive treatment, the cost will probably run from $2,000 to $3,000. If a patient requires extensive reconstructive work as part of Phase II, the cost can be much much higher. There is no way around stating that TMJ treatment can be costly.

INSURANCE COVERAGE

Insurance coverage for TMJ is variable. People with standard health insurance coverage can have an appendectomy

113

and expect the insurance company to cover this procedure. It is considered standard and therefore will not be challenged. TMJ treatment is handled differently for many reasons, some having to do with the nature of the disorder.

TMJ is a dentally based orthopedic disorder with medical manifestations. The basic source of the problem might be the teeth, but the symptoms mimic many medical disorders and complaints. Numerous branches of the healing arts are called upon to treat headaches, neck, shoulder, and back pain. Even bruxing is often viewed not as a dental problem, but as a psychological one.

Many patients believe that their dental insurance will be an appropriate source of coverage for TMJ treatment. However, this is seldom true for Phase I treatment. Dental insurance usually covers dental surgical procedures, such as fillings and root canals. Dental policies often limit the amount paid per year per family member. They may exclude orthodontia or other procedures having to do with occlusal changes (changes in the way the teeth fit together when the mouth closes).

Because TMJ is on the borderline between medical and dental concerns, some medical insurers don't want to deal with it. To them, it sounds like dental procedures and, therefore, outside the realm of medical coverage.

Because of all these dilemmas, insurance coverage for TMJ can be sporadic and unpredictable. Sometimes medical insurance covers Phase I treatment, and then dental insurance picks up portions of Phase II treatment.

MEDICAL POLICIES

It makes sense for medical insurance, which usually covers orthopedic procedures, to cover Phase I treatment, basically because the splint is an orthopedic appliance. It allows the jaw to move and function normally. Also, treatment in Phase I is eliminating symptoms that have medical implications.

To date, many medical insurance companies pay benefits for TMJ therapy. However, more and more insurance companies are adding TMJ treatment to their exclusion riders. Because diagnosis of TMJ is becoming more common, companies are making these decisions in order to keep total costs down. Some policies do offer TMJ treatment inclusion as a special option.

If you are considering treatment for TMJ, examine your policy and see whether the condition is specifically mentioned. If it is excluded, you will not be covered for nonsurgical treatment for TMJ. Most exclusion riders state that surgical intervention into the joint will be covered. Since only 2 to 5 percent of the patients seeking treatment for the condition need surgery, this has serious implications. It encourages people to seek the kind of treatment their policies cover, rather than what is most appropriate and safe.

The kinds of coverage people receive from their medical policies vary, too. Some policies cover the splint but not the needle puncture. Others cover the needle puncture but not the splint. This is handled on a case-by-case basis and is still unpredictable.

THE INSURANCE DILEMMA

The insurance dilemma is one that needs to be resolved in order to provide coverage for this common and often debilitating disorder. Not covering TMJ makes little sense, considering that the costs of investigation into the cause of headaches often are covered. Some patients whose insurance companies have paid thousands and thousands of dollars for tests, examinations, and treatments have never gotten better. Now that an effective treatment is available for the cause of so much pain, it seems ridiculous not to cover it. In the long run, much money could be saved.

When people are looking at insurance options, they should consider which kind of policy will have the best options for TMJ. Sometimes it means paying an extra premium to have the treatment included. For other people it means choosing an insurance plan rather than joining an HMO or a capitation plan. A capitation plan may be fine if the group of dentists being contracted with includes a dentist who can do successful TMJ treatment. Since few HMOs include dentistry, coverage for TMJ treatment, except surgery, is unavailable.

Many patients end up paying large portions of the treatment costs themselves. Often they do this because they see the treatment as an investment in their future. Numerous patients have been able to live fuller and more productive lives after they had TMJ treatment. Pain takes an enormous toll, and few people who live in chronic pain are able to manage highly successful careers. But once they become pain-free and can live normally, they realize their personal potentials. Patients have told me that in the long run the treatment much more than paid for itself through advancement in business or a career that became possible when TMJ was resolved. In fact most have said that it was the best investment they had ever made.

In the coming years, there will be many changes in insurance company policy regarding TMJ treatment. This is bound to happen as more and more people seek help and raise questions about coverage. Changes will also occur because the condition is becoming more widely known and recognized in the health care community. But at this time do not *assume* that treatment will be covered. Choose your insurance plan cautiously.

13

After TMJ Treatment

I appreciate life more than most people I know. I didn't have a life before.   —a 34-year-old musician

It's like starting all over again. But it's exciting.
     —a 40-year-old psychotherapist

Many patients enter TMJ therapy doubting that they will ever be pain-free. One patient had been through two surgeries, a year of orthodontia, a year of wearing a splint, and physical therapy. "Whatever you do, it will only last two weeks," she said. However, she did agree to start TMJ therapy again, even though she was convinced that it would benefit her for only two weeks. After about eight weeks of Phase I treatment, she was symptom-free for about sixteen consecutive days; after that, her progress was rapid. When she was finally convinced that her life could be pain-free, she said, "I think I'll make plans for three weeks from now."

In a nutshell, the biggest change many TMJ patients experience is being able to plan life more than one day ahead. Many have become used to thinking about work and play in terms of the pain they are in, or may be in. When they no longer have to consider the pain in their plans, an enormous burden is lifted. Many are so accustomed to that burden that they have forgotten what it was like to live in freedom from constant pain.

Patients who are beginning recovery in Phase I often complain about having to come in for weekly visits. Some will comment on the difference in their attitude. "I was so glad to get here when we first started," one patient said. "But now it's such a bother. I'm too busy catching up with my life."

REFUTING STEREOTYPES

Many stereotypes exist about people in pain—they are hypochondriacs, they use pain to control people, they are in pain because they are depressed, they need the pain as a way to avoid responsibility. Certainly these stereotypes may apply to some people. A minute number of patients have had some kind of need to have the pain. But in the eighteen years I have been treating TMJ these people have been so few that I can barely remember them.

Remember Sandy Gilbert? Her husband carried a beeper so that she could reach him. She often had to call him to come and rescue her when a headache struck. Most of the people who knew her, except her husband, believed she was trying to control her husband with pain.

About two months into treatment, Ms. Gilbert told her husband to throw the beeper away. "It was the happiest day of my life," she said. "I hated the beeper, and I hated what people were saying about me." For Ms. Gilbert, a new life opened up when she was pain-free. She began spending time with her daughters and grandchildren. "We went shopping for a whole day, and I didn't think about pain once," she said. "I haven't done that for years. Even holidays were planned around 'mother's condition,' and the family got tired of it."

Sarah Johnson started looking for a teaching job as soon as her treatment was over. "Imagine. I was worried that I really was depressed. Now I know that it was truly the pain that finally got me down," she said. Ms. Johnson had been through so much that it would have been normal for her to have a long reentry period. However, that was not the case. She typifies many patients who have lived in agonizing pain. When the pain is over, they jump back into life—usually with both feet.

REBUILDING MARRIAGES AND LIVES

Some patients have experienced destroyed marriages. In a sense they have a double tragedy. They have lived in physical pain, and also had a spouse who either couldn't understand what they were going through or couldn't live with the problems. This is perfectly understandable. Living with a person in chronic pain means living a "handicapped" life as well.

Ray Foreman had to rebuild almost everything in his life. He'd lost his wife, his social life, and a successful business. Mr. Foreman began psychotherapy during treatment. "I think I am in a depression," he said. "I've lost a lot, and I want help getting some of it back." He felt an enormous amount of anger toward his ex-wife, and while he couldn't recapture that relationship, he was able to be on friendly terms with her after he had some help.

A patient like Mr. Foreman literally has to rebuild everything. Often a patient like this can benefit from some kind of psychological counseling. He knew the depression wasn't causing his pain, because his pain was gone by the time he began to get help for the depression. It took him almost two years to rebuild a social life, start another business, and, in short, live normally. "I was so isolated that I felt like I had to become a 'social animal' all over again. I was uncomfortable with people for quite a while," he said.

Another patient had given custody of her child to her ex-husband. After treatment was complete, she was able to negotiate joint custody of their son, an arrangement agreeable to the father. "He wasn't being vindictive when he took custody," she explained. "I was unable to take care of him. He's relieved too that I'm well enough to take care of our child." The kind of relief and joy a patient like this feels is almost impossible to describe.

SMALLER CHANGES

Most patients' recovery isn't that dramatic. Many patients notice smaller things—an ability to sleep well is a common one. If sleep has been disturbed by pain, the patient often adjusts to the disturbance and may not even mention it during the initial evaluation. But a month or two into treatment, the patient may say, "I can sleep so much better than I used to. I just noticed this."

Sometimes patients begin doing things they couldn't do before treatment. Joy Rubin, the patient with restricted neck motion, had at one time been an avid tennis player. One of the first things she did was dust off her racket and get back to the courts. Former runners go back to the track, and weight lifters go back to the gym. The patients are asked to resume these activities slowly in case symptoms are retriggered. It's important always to treat the jaw mechanism carefully, because we know that these muscles are vulnerable to spasm.

Sometimes patients have to be cautioned against trying to do too many things at once. Some patients want to take up two or three physical activities immediately, when they really should add activities one at a time. If for some reason symptoms are retriggered by weight lifting, jogging, or scuba diving, it's better to be able to isolate the activity. The chances of retriggering TMJ symptoms are slim, but muscles that have been in spasm should be treated with some caution. This is especially true during attempts to solve the problem permanently in Phase II. During Phase II, spasms may be triggered inadvertently either by physical activity or by stressing the jaw during the dental treatment itself.

FUTURE DENTAL AND MEDICAL CARE

Once a TMJ patient has had treatment, any future dental work needs to be carried out according to the concepts underlying the Phase II definitive work. Dentists need to be aware of the delicate gearing scheme created and that it was done with special care to avoid stressing the jaw. Dental work can retrigger TMJ symptoms.

In patients with combination headaches, once the TMJ component has been taken care of, the patient can go on to have further diagnostic evaluations and treatment. In the case of a patient who is being treated for allergies, the search for "forbidden" food becomes much easier. A patient who suspected an allergy to dairy products found out that she truly was sensitive to that family of foods. The coming and going of TMJ symptoms had stopped, and gradually it became possible to test more foods. Some were removed and others reintroduced into her diet.

Many patients suffering from true migraines notice having fewer of them after TMJ treatment. Although it's unclear why TMJ headaches trigger other kinds, this phenomenon occurs over and over. Patients who are sensitive to chemicals commonly found in foods—MSG or preservatives, for example—can see patterns, and cause and effect, in their headaches. Before the TMJ component was removed, isolating causes was often much too confusing.

Patients who have used many self-help techniques often continue them or discontinue them based on how much the techniques have enhanced their lives overall. People who have taken up yoga, meditation, massage, or exercise programs often keep them up because they find them enjoyable and beneficial in other ways. Sometimes they find they get more pleasure from the activities when they view these measures as optional rather than mandatory. "I was down on myself if I missed a relaxation class," one woman said. "I felt so responsible for my own pain."

We also warn patients about surgical treatment after TMJ treatment. Sometimes surgery can trigger TMJ in the first place because of the tube that is passed into the windpipe when the patient is under general anesthesia. This tube takes over the patient's breathing during the surgery. However, for the tube to be passed down the patient's throat, his or her mouth must be opened very wide. The patient is unconscious and can't tell the physicians that his or her jaw is being stretched too wide and is being stressed.

Generally the same function can be served by using a nasal-tracheal tube. This involves passing the tube down the patient's nose, into the throat, and on to the windpipe. The anesthesiologist opens the patient's mouth briefly to see where the tube is going, but the stress is for a much shorter period of time.

When a patient who has had TMJ treatment is going to have surgery, a nasal tube should be used rather than an oral tube. Most physicians are cooperative once they understand the reason for the request. The problem is seldom insurmountable. However, the patient should remember to discuss this with the physician. Sometimes people want to put their experience with TMJ so far behind them that they forget to consider their past vulnerability to muscle spasm.

RENEWED LIFE

Some routine observations about post-TMJ patients haven't been scientifically documented. More research may make it possible to quantify some effects of pain and its removal. Many patients have reported an overall improvement in their well-being. They sleep better and have fewer colds, many report eating better, and some say they have less indigestion or other digestive disturbances.

Nearly every person who sought treatment because of debilitating pain reports having more energy after treatment. Pain can be exhausting, and patients seldom realize how exhausting until it's gone and they feel their normal energy return. Patients have said they have tried new things—sports, night classes, new careers, or having babies they had put off having because they didn't feel they could handle parental responsibility while in pain. And some patients establish relationships and marriages they felt they couldn't handle because of incapacitating pain.

Even patients whose symptoms and life losses were less severe report having increased energy and ability to live fully. Their new lease on life may be less dramatic, but they still mention them throughout treatment and after. Patients with less severe symptoms often say that they had become used to living at an unnecessarily slow pace.

Patients who are lucky enough to have supportive family members, spouses, and friends report a kind of renewal. They routinely say things like, "My sense of humor is back. We joke more now in our house. People aren't so careful not to disturb me for fear of being snapped at." Others will say that their sexual lives are more normal, too. "It was a relief to know that I really did a have a normal sex drive—it was just pain that got in the way," one man said. The "not tonight, dear" joke has often been attributed to women, but anyone who treats TMJ knows that men, too, are unable to enjoy normal sex lives when pain takes over.

Some patients are able to take care of other health concerns now that the pain is out of the way. For instance, I've seen patients deal with weight problems they couldn't handle before. Other patients take up much-needed exercise programs for the first time. Pain had prevented them from doing almost any physical activity, even though they had been advised to start an exercise program as part of a treatment for high blood pressure or heart disease.

In general the life of the ex-TMJ patient is pleasant indeed. For a few people who were long-term TMJ sufferers, it seems as if they are beginning life for the first time. These people, as well as some shorter-term sufferers, even look different. Their faces are more relaxed, they smile more, and their eyes are brighter.

14
Guidelines for Seeking Help

*Gradually I realized that pain had taken over my life—
feeling it, thinking about it, and trying to get rid of it.*
                                        —a 24-year-old teacher

Will I have to live like this forever?
                                        —a 52-year-old carpenter

TMJ is not life-threatening, nor does it cause
progressive physical damage. That is to say, it hasn't been
conclusively shown that TMJ does progressive damage. As
more is learned about TMJ, and research is compiled, we
may discover long-term physical changes. But, as far as we
now know, none exist. Also, patients occasionally become
suicidal because of the pain they suffer, and some lives are
all but destroyed by pain. In that sense, TMJ can indeed
threaten the life of a person whose pain becomes unbearable, but TMJ itself does not directly threaten the sufferer's
life.

Because TMJ is a pain syndrome and not degenerative or
life-threatening, the necessity for treatment usually depends
on the patient's desires and degree of discomfort. Often in
the course of a dental examination, patients reveal symptoms of TMJ. They may have occasional headaches or neck
and shoulder aches, but they consider these to be minor
episodes and not disruptive to their daily lives. Many
patients have daily headaches that are mild and relieved by

over-the-counter pain killers. These headaches are not interfering with the patient's life, and he or she has accommodated them. Therefore, treatment isn't indicated. Other people with a similar quantity and quality of symptoms desire treatment for the problem. The differentiating feature is the individual's response to the pain.

REASONS FOR SEEKING CARE

Pain is usually the motivating factor in seeking help. Treatment is also advisable if a patient is going to begin sophisticated dental procedures such as reconstructive work, bridges, or multiple crowns. This is advisable whether or not the patient is exhibiting symptoms. Remember that the symptoms of TMJ may be triggered or worsened by extensive dental treatment when that individual has a predisposition to the problem—a tooth-gearing problem and muscle spasms. This is true even in a patient without symptoms. Many times, the first TMJ symptoms a person experiences occur after extensive dental treatment.

Any person who is currently taking medication for headaches or any other symptoms commonly seen in TMJ should find out the diagnosis of the problem and the purpose of the medication. If the diagnosis is merely descriptive or the purpose of the medication is simply to mask the pain, then evaluation for TMJ is desirable.

Remember: Pain is a result of processes occurring in the body that are potentially harmful to a person's well-being. Pain is not a disease in itself. If the reason for the pain can be corrected, the pain will cease. This is what happens in TMJ treatment. It follows that when the patient's pain is gone, he or she need not rely on body- and mind-numbing medications that at best can only mask the discomfort. In addition, these medications aren't always effective with TMJ pain anyway.

Treatment whose only effect is the relief of pain through medication ignores one simple fact: *All pain has a reason.* But unfortunately, all the health care professions combined haven't uncovered all the reasons yet. Nor is it practical to assume that each individual practitioner can possibly be aware of all the known reasons for pain.

Medication for pain may be beneficial when it's impossible to determine the reason for pain, or the pain can't be dealt with in any other way—for example, after surgery or a tooth extraction. However, a great many patients who have sought TMJ treatment had been told repeatedly that there was no reason for their pain. They often are taking large quantities of pain-relief medication to mask their symptoms.

Frequently the reason for their pain is TMJ. It's usually possible to treat the condition and eliminate the pain. Before successful TMJ treatment was available, attempting to mask the pain was the only choice. But fortunately, that is not the case today.

EVALUATING CARE

With the practitioner you see, explore and discuss the many different approaches used for TMJ treatment. I can only take responsibility for, and speak knowledgeably about, the treatment techniques I have developed and have discussed in this book. I use these techniques daily in my practice, and they have successfully resolved my patients' problems in most cases. Because I cannot make specific judgments about other techniques, you will have to weigh this book's suggestions about what to be aware of when seeking TMJ treatment, along with the advice of the practitioner you are consulting.

SURGERY OR OTHER DEFINITIVE TREATMENT

Many people who have had TMJ treatment still have pain. In the course of treatment, many have had major oral alterations, such as orthodontics, tooth movement, surgery on the temporomandibular joint, jaw surgery, and equilibration. The definitive (Phase II) treatment described in this book is usually considered *only* after the patient is symptom-free. No one can offer a "treatment guarantee," but if Phase I treatment is unsuccessful, the definitive treatment has little chance of succeeding.

Generally, definitive treatment should be considered after three things happen:

1. The symptoms—pain and distress—are eliminated.
2. The signs—muscle spasms, for example—that the practitioner sees are eliminated.
3. The movement of the lower jaw toward its normal position has stopped.

Although the patient usually begins to feel significantly improved in one to three weeks, the course of Phase I treatment may last for several months. Even when there is demonstrable damage to the jaw, if the patient exhibits muscle spasms, we will treat the patient muscularly in Phase I. If the patient doesn't respond to treatment in a reasonable period of time, we will then make an exception in our protocol and refer the patient for evaluation and possible surgery of the joint itself.

PART-TIME USE OF THE SPLINT

When a splint is worn only part-time, the likelihood of lasting success or success at all drastically diminishes. This is only logical. The triggering mechanism for TMJ is a problem twenty-four hours a day, and it is not under the patient's conscious control. Any device designed to eliminate the triggering mechanism will have maximum effectiveness only if used full-time. When the device is out of the mouth, the bite-triggering mechanism has full effect and may even be enhanced. This occurs because the muscles have begun to relax and have started to "forget" their protective role.

Most patients accept wearing the splint full-time as a temporary and small hardship compared to the pain they've been in. If the patient can't wear the splint twenty-four hours a day, then treatment should generally not be considered at that time. The chances of success are minute, and wastes the patient's money and the practitioner's time.

FREQUENT AND ROUTINE OFFICE VISITS

In an effective treatment protocol, it is vital to see patients regularly, usually weekly, during Phase I. As mentioned, this treatment phase involves forcible relaxation of the muscles and adjustment of the splint to accommodate the new position of the jaw. When office visits are spaced more widely than once a week, patients tend to progress more slowly. They also have more pain, and the treatment is longer and less predictable. Be specifically aware of the frequency of these all-important visits.

HEAVY USE OF DRUG THERAPY

Pain-relief medication should not be necessary during TMJ treatment. Usually within the first weeks of treatment, patients experience substantial relief. In addition, multiple therapies tend to confuse both the practitioner and the patient. If symptoms and signs change, it's difficult to determine which approach was responsible for the changes. An additional and equally important reason for not using drug therapy is that it's most often ineffective, and patients obtain rapid relief without it. Thus, it's unnecessary.

TREATMENT TIME

It's unfortunate but true that many patients recite a history of years of therapy without results. Treatment time varies, and it depends on the patient's response to therapy. This is impossible to predict, but patients typically respond positively within a month—generally within the first three weeks. On the average, Phase I treatment lasts four to six months.

TMJ treatment has a beginning and an end. It is *not* a lifelong maintenance treatment. The first goal of treatment is to eliminate the problem by artificial means. When this is done, changes are made in the patient's mouth so that the accomplishments of Phase I can be maintained without treatment devices. *You should not be a TMJ patient forever.*

TREATMENT TECHNIQUES

Many common techniques have been shown to be of some value in treating TMJ patients and are used by some practitioners. Some of these techniques are logical, since TMJ is both a pain syndrome and related to stress. These techniques are not bad in and of themselves, and some may help particular patients more effectively deal with stress in their lives. Some therapies help patients handle their pain.

However, they do not help the *underlying reason* for TMJ symptoms, and therefore are seldom used to treat patients in my office. But readers of this book may encounter practitioners who do incorporate them in their philosophies of TMJ therapy.

MOIST-HEAT THERAPY

Moist-heat therapy is sometimes used as a self-help measure and is useful for home care. Some office treatment uses this as well. It generally involves applying moist hot towels or special devices to the head, face, and neck. The goal of the treatment is to relieve pain by breaking the muscle-spasm cycle. In this case, the heat becomes the irritant to the muscle. It also stimulates circulation to the area and may reduce inflammation.

Before the development of the muscle-puncture technique, which is fast and predictable, the moist-heat treatment was certainly an efficacious therapy to use. However, the needle-puncture technique breaks spasms and relaxes the muscles so effectively that the heat treatment is no longer necessary.

CRYOTHERAPY

Cryotherapy is an old technique that is sometimes effective in preventing the spread of a headache. When used in the office, a medication called ethyl chloride is sprayed on the skin. This medication evaporates rapidly and chills the surface on which it is sprayed. A more simple technique involves putting a cold pack on the head, face, or neck when the headache first begins. A cold pack works most effectively on vascular headaches and has not been found specifically effective in stopping the spread of muscular headaches. But this technique helps occasionally. Again, the cold may serve as the muscle irritant and break the spasm.

TRANSCUTANEOUS ELECTRO-NEURAL STIMULATION (TENS)

With TENS, electrodes connected to a portable battery pack are applied to the tender areas, possibly suppressing pain in those places. The apparent action of TENS is to interfere with the sensation of pain. It doesn't take away the cause of pain, but acts to block the message of pain to the brain. There is some evidence to suggest that TENS stimulates the release of endorphins, the body's natural narcotic. This mechanism may provide some relief temporarily. In TMJ this relief is unusually unpredictable.

Now that it is known how accessible the key muscles are in TMJ treatment, and how easily we can relax them, TENS is neither necessary nor beneficial to TMJ patients. However, in the treatment of other pain syndromes, TENS may be very effective and the most practical way to reduce symptoms.

ELECTRICALLY STIMULATING THE MUSCLES OF MASTICATION

Electrical stimulation of the muscles of mastication is a technique similar to TENS, but it doesn't suppress pain directly. Its apparent action is to control the muscle spasms in the muscles of mastication by stimulating facial nerves. The concept of this treatment is that muscles may relax as a result of increased blood flow. This may indeed happen, but it takes longer, uses a more expensive technology, and is less predictable than the simple muscle-puncture method.

Therefore, it isn't necessary in TMJ treatment.

HIGH-VOLTAGE ELECTRO-GALVANIC STIMULATION

The goal of high-voltage electro-galvanic stimulation is to reduce muscle spasms and pain by applying a certain type of electricity to various muscles. Its goal is similar to that of the needle-puncture technique. The needle-puncture technique is usually more comfortable for the patient, however, and the results are faster and more predictable.

ULTRASOUND THERAPY

Ultrasound therapy enables heat to reach areas that can't be treated topically. It may reduce symptoms temporarily, but it doesn't treat the cause of pain. Use of this kind of device may increase the cost of therapy simply because the technology is more expensive than the syringes used in the needle-puncture technique. Ultrasound therapy is also less predictable, and muscle relaxation takes longer to achieve.

DIGITAL STETHOSCOPE

The term *Doppler-effect technology* is used to describe the development of technology that enables a practitioner to hear through tissues in the body. It was originally developed to monitor fetal heartbeat and later became used in assessing the functioning of artificial heart valves. This same technology is used in a type of stethoscope that enables practitioners to classify sounds the temporomandibular joint makes upon opening and closing. Currently, several researchers are trying to correlate data from the digital stethoscope with various types of joint derangements.

This instrument shows much promise for learning what is happening inside the joint. It may give oral surgeons a better picture of what they will find when they enter surgically.

At the present time, the digital stethoscope has questionable value for use in TMJ treatment. Even when a patient has joint derangement, the pain is most often caused by muscle spasms, and treatment goals are usually achieved without surgery. The digital stethoscope may be useful to the oral surgeon when surgery on the joint is deemed necessary.

THERAPEUTIC EXERCISES

Some practitioners try to treat TMJ by retraining certain muscles and/or the tongue. Sometimes the therapy includes exercises that correct the position of the tongue and help balance the facial muscles and the muscles of mastication while in use. The exercises also attempt to relieve muscle spasms. However, I have found that most exercises of this type impede rather than aid the patient. On rare occasions, certain exercises may be necessary during Phase II of treatment, but they by no means should be part of a routine treatment plan.

BIOFEEDBACK

Biofeedback is a well-known technique for treatment of pain and stress syndromes. Patients learn to control muscle contraction by monitoring various body signals, thereby attempting to relax sufficiently to stop the pain cycle. Electronic instruments are used to indicate to the patient when the muscles are contracting. This feedback mechanism helps patients make a conscious effort to relax the muscles. Over time, patients can use the information when they are not working with the machine, enabling them to relax for longer periods of time. Some people find the monitoring of relaxation very stressful in itself; others have found the technique helpful in showing them ways to consciously attain a relaxed state.

Biofeedback was once thought to be a panacea for chronic pain syndromes. However, TMJ has a physiologic trigger that is present twenty-four hours a day, and that may produce symptoms at any time, whether a patient is relaxed or not. Furthermore, if the *cause* of pain is eliminated, it is not necessary to help patients learn how to cope with the pain.

STRESS MANAGEMENT AND PSYCHOTHERAPY

A case can be made that every person, with or without TMJ problems, can benefit from training in stress management. Many TMJ patients have difficulty relaxing and will describe themselves as "tense" individuals. We know stress is a component in TMJ as well as in many other disorders. The stress of having chronic TMJ symptoms will often leave a patient vulnerable to other health problems because of lowered resistance. Stress can also exacerbate existing conditions such as high blood pressure. It makes sense for all of us to learn how to deal with the inevitable stresses in our lives and learn how to relax.

Many people, including some TMJ patients, have difficulties in their lives that cause them to seek psychotherapy. Some TMJ patients have sought therapy after completing treatment because they wanted help in putting their devastated lives back in order. Chronic pain sufferers often lead empty lives when pain destroys, or all but destroys, any chance for normalcy. Patients' family lives, careers, relationships, and leisure activities become ruled by pain. Some patients are able to rise above the pain and manage to carry on a facade of normal life. Others become vegetables because of medications, and they often lose their ability to be involved with other people and in social activities. And, of course, many patients work out in psychotherapy problems that have nothing whatsoever to do with TMJ.

While psychotherapy can benefit individuals for many reasons, I don't often recommend it *as part of TMJ treatment*. My treatment for TMJ corrects a physiologic trigger for pain and relaxes the muscles. It doesn't teach patients to cope with the pain, rise above pain, or numb pain with drugs. It eliminates the cause of the pain itself.

SOME RECOMMENDATIONS

Because of my treatment approach, I can't advocate or advise patients to seek the other therapies I've listed here—except in rare instances. In fact, in the first months of therapy patients are advised to stop all other measures they have been taking to help them with TMJ—chiropractic, physical therapy, massage, whatever. Of course, if a patient is already in psychotherapy, they aren't asked to stop seeing the therapist. If they have been practicing transcendental meditation for years, they can continue. But they are asked not to begin any new therapies.

When this treatment approach is the only recent change in the patient's life and the patient is improving, it is logical to assume that he or she is getting better because of that change. Using these other therapies, especially at the beginning of treatment, would make it impossible to know which therapies are causing which effects. The treatment approach outlined in this book is predictable. If a patient isn't starting to improve within a month, treatment is usually discontinued. At that point, we reevaluate the likelihood of success if we continue or change the treatment regimen. We usually conclude the chances are slim, and the patient is referred to other specialists.

Anyone who is seeking help for TMJ, or even seeking evaluation and diagnosis, should look for a practitioner who can treat the cause of the problem. Because TMJ should not require lifelong maintenance therapy, and because therapy should have a beginning, a middle, and—most important—an end, find out the reasons for the therapy you choose, and its end.

If you suffer from regular TMJ symptoms, I urge you to find a competent practitioner whose experience shows that TMJ can be corrected with well-thought-out and methodical treatment.

15
Self-Help

I don't want headaches to drive me to the couch. I'd like to live a normal life—work, play, eat, and sleep. I don't want to think about pain every minute. —a 51-year-old lawyer

My life became a cycle of trying to avoid pain, and failing at that too often, I spent my time getting rid of the pain. It was a hellish life. —a 30-year-old nurse

        Some people with mild to moderate TMJ symptoms are able to help themselves prevent or manage pain or discomfort. Unfortunately, self-help measures are totally successful in only a minority of cases. People who seek various "home remedies" or self-administered pain-relief techniques usually have already sought help from health care professionals. Often they have been unable to obtain help; many were given descriptive diagnoses, rather than diagnoses linked to the cause of the problem. When the cause of pain can't be detected, the patient is often left alone to cope.

    Some people who have attempted self-help have been given a diagnosis of TMJ, but for any number of reasons— including financial concerns, other health problems that take priority, or geographical location—do not seek treatment to get rid of the cause of their pain. Many people with TMJ experience symptoms erratically. They go along year after year, having temporary bouts with pain, and manage to cope. Since TMJ is not life-threatening, the decision to seek treatment is private and personal. Those who suffer minor and infrequent symptoms often feel, reasonably, that their problem is not serious enough to warrant treatment at that time. But at least they know that a permanent solution to their problems is available if symptoms worsen.

People who do not choose treatment often wonder what they can do for themselves to attempt to prevent or relieve TMJ symptoms. The suggestions given here may work in *particular* cases. If they don't prevent or relieve symptoms, then you are one of the majority. This is important to remember. Patients often feel that if self-help measures don't work, TMJ isn't really their problem; they even may believe that the pain is of psychological origin. This only adds to their stress. Give these suggestions a try if you wish, but do not fall into the trap of believing there is no reason for your pain. The secret of success in treating pain syndromes is proper diagnosis.

PAIN KILLERS

It's certainly logical for people to try over-the-counter pain relievers for minor problems. It's important to remember that aspirin, acetaminophen, and ibuprofen may mask minor symptoms, but will not cure the real problem. These pain relievers just raise the person's threshold for being bothered by the discomfort.

Those who do find relief with over-the-counter pain killers usually find they're most effective if taken when the pain first starts. However, for most people with other than very mild TMJ symptoms, this self-help measure is of little use. Most patients report that they take them more out of hope that they will get some relief rather than from the experience of finding help through them. One patient said, "The chances of any pain relievers working are about one in ten, but I try them despite the odds."

It's a common—but not advisable—practice to keep left-over prescription pain relievers in the home medicine cabinet. Patients have commented that these rarely are of any use. In general, neither over-the-counter nor prescription drugs are particularly helpful for TMJ symptoms.

KEEPING THE TEETH APART

TMJ-related muscles spasms are triggered when the teeth touch each other or are ground together in an abnormal gearing relationship. Consequently, one of the most important home prevention methods is to avoid letting your teeth touch each other. This is much easier said than done, however. The teeth close every time you swallow, and the swallowing reflex occurs about 2,000 times a day. Teeth also naturally touch when you are under stress, or when you pick up something heavy.

Although it is possible to consciously try to keep the teeth apart during the day just by using willpower, many TMJ sufferers find an "artificial" method helpful. If you want to try this method, take a small cotton ball, or cotton roll like those used in dentistry, or a tightly rolled piece of tissue, and hold it between your teeth on one side. You can use your tongue and cheek to keep the cotton ball or tissue from falling off the biting surfaces of the teeth.

It might seem that the purpose of the ball in this location is to physically keep the teeth from touching. Actually, its purpose is to let you know when your teeth are beginning to close down on each other. It feels unusual to try to close the teeth when there is an obstruction. This feeling triggers awareness, and when this technique is successful, the user is often able to keep the teeth apart a significant portion of the day.

This technique may sound impractical. It takes some practice and perseverence, but it is actually one of the most effective self-help techniques available. People who use it trade off a dry feeling in their mouths for relief or prevention. They also learn to work and concentrate with a foreign object in their mouths. Sometimes people report that the tissue dissolves quickly. This happens when the tissue isn't tightly rolled.

Some years ago a patient who didn't want to pursue treatment at the time of diagnosis tried this technique. She found it impractical for herself, because she couldn't work with the public in her sales job with a mouth full of cotton. However, she suggested it to her husband, a computer programmer, who experienced a headache every afternoon. He attributed his headaches to the stress of deadlines and the intense concentration his work required. He found the cotton-roll technique helpful because he could avoid clenching his teeth as the pressure of the day built.

Because he found the technique so successful, he told others in the office about it. Before long, the company nurse noticed a steady stream of workers coming in after lunch asking for cotton rolls. She became curious about the reasons for the run on the cotton-roll supply, and her investigation eventuallly led her to call my office. Her response to my explanation was, "It must work, because I'm having fewer requests for aspirin."

This self-help technique became a company joke, and those who used it were the objects of much teasing. Other people, not familiar with the strain of regular headaches, couldn't understand how anyone could tolerate such an inconvenience. Only those who understand this kind of pain know that in this case anyway, the prevention is much more convenient than tolerating the discomfort of a headache.

Warning: This technique **must not be used during sleeping hours**, because there is a great danger that the cotton ball, tissue, or other home device will be either swallowed accidentally, or drawn into the lungs or air passages connecting the lungs. These are extremely dangerous situations. **Do not use** this technique any time you have a condition that suppresses your cough or gag reflex, or when exercising strenuously. Also **do not use** it when there is even a slight possibility of dozing or losing alertness, as when drinking alcohol, using any drug, watching television, or lying down to relax. Use this technique **only** when you are going about routine activities fully awake, alert, and aware.

The cotton-ball or tissue technique may be successful during the day, but because of the danger involved, keeping the teeth from touching is a much more difficult problem during the night. The best technique, and perhaps the only one with some success at night, is simply to sleep on your back with a small pillow beneath your neck. Your neck arches and extends your head backward. Before you try it, ask your phsycian if there is any reason this sleeping position is inappropriate for you. Unfortunately, most people find this position nearly impossible, because they naturally and unconsciously move to their sides and stomachs during the night.

It may seem surprising that sleeping position is related to TMJ problems, but picture the body in various sleeping postures. Except when you sleep on your back, your jaw must rest on something—your arm, the pillow, or the mattress. This can push the teeth together, and may also force the jaw into an abnormal and strained position.

Using an artificial method during the day—the tissue or cotton ball—and sleeping on your back at night *may* help prevent the onset of symptoms or relieve them should they occur. This applies to all the TMJ symptoms, not just headaches. Virtually all TMJ symptoms are the result of the teeth touching in an abnormal gearing scheme. The resulting muscle spasms produce the complement of symptoms discussed in this book, including extremity numbness, middle-ear symptoms, and shoulder pain.

BREAKING HABITS

Some common habits can contribute to TMJ problems. Most people aren't aware that these habits can exacerbate symptoms or trigger them in the first place.

Anyone with a susceptibility to TMJ problems should avoid chewing gum. It can create problems in two ways. First, it tends to overwork the very muscles causing the pain. In the process of chewing gum, the teeth generally do not touch each other directly. This tends to trick the neuromuscular system into relaxing, making the system vulnerable to the spasm-triggering mechanism or the still-present gearing problem when the gum is no longer in the mouth.

Many patients have complained about experiencing almost constant headaches that began after they stopped smoking cigarettes. They started to chew gum to help themselves cope with the withdrawal period. Most patients first attributed these headaches to nicotine withdrawal, then realized that this was not the case, since the headaches didn't go away in a short period of time. Rather, the gum chewing itself became a habit, and the constant movement of the jaw plus the "tricking" of the neuromuscular system brought on TMJ symptoms. Breaking the gum-chewing habit was enough to relieve symptoms in many of these patients.

Other small, often unconscious habits may contribute to TMJ problems. Chewing on pens or pencils is one example. One patient said this habit was as hard to break as giving up cigarettes, but once she did, the frequency and severity of her symptoms declined. Chewing and clamping down on pipes and cigars can have the same unbalancing effect on the jaw. When the jaw is out of balance, the temporomandibular joint is stressed, possibly triggering symptoms.

If you have any of the symptoms of TMJ—even mild ones—try to be more conscious of how many times you rest your head, chin, or jaw on the heel of your hands. The jaw sits on your hands in a position that can add to the pressure on your teeth and then trigger the pain mechanism. Curbing this habit can help, although patients report that it's difficult to do.

TELEPHONE USE

The telephone, a tool we consider indispensable in modern life, can also greatly contribute to TMJ problems. This occurs when the receiver is held between the shoulder and the ear in order to free both hands. In this position, the telephone rests on, and stresses, the lower jaw. This unnatural pressure may trigger TMJ problems. The neck muscles are also strained, and this may exacerbate the muscle spasms.

Unfortunately, there are devices available that aid in and promote this cradling position and contribute to TMJ problems in susceptible people. Probably no major problems will result from cradling a telephone receiver with or without a device, for a minute or two once in a while. However, some people use these devices to extremes. Distorting the position of, and putting pressure on, the lower jaw, head, and neck significantly contribute to TMJ problems.

Fortunately for people who must use the telephone with both hands free, the cradling problem is easily solved without adding strain on the head, neck, and jaw. Speaker telephones, which don't even need to be held, are now widely available. Another helpful device is a headset similar to those used by telephone operators and pilots. These lightweight headsets do not put any strain on the muscles in the head and neck, nor do they stress the jaw.

DIET

Eating foods with certain textures may trigger or worsen TMJ symptoms. Hard, crunchy foods like Corn Nuts or hard candy or chewy caramels can be extremely stressful to the jaw. Chewing on ice can have the same effect. A few foods have mixed consistencies and the jaw is "tricked" into thinking the food is soft. Because the jaw is confused, it doesn't protect itself against the hard pieces of food that are mixed with the soft; the jaw is "surprised" when it encounters them, and muscle spasms may be triggered. An example of this is a walnut or a shell inside a soft cookie. A small piece of bone in a hamburger is another example, and these situations can be significant triggers for TMJ symptoms.

The pressures and unbalancing effects on the jaw necessary to break apart hard foods can stress the temporomandibular joint, and the neuromuscular system may respond to the stress by triggering spasms. Additionally, the teeth and fillings may be damaged by the force of the confused jaw mechanism.

Eliminating hard foods is often advisable for TMJ sufferers because it gives the jaw mechanism a chance to rest. There is a literal rule of thumb advisable for TMJ patients: They should open their mouths no wider than necessary to accommodate a thumb.

STRESS MANAGEMENT

Many people try to reduce their symptoms through stress-reduction techniques. Physical exercise is one of the most widely accepted ways to handle stress, yet many types of exercise will increase the tendency to clamp down on the teeth or tighten the jaw. Bicycle riding, jogging, weightlifting, using exercise equipment, aerobic dancing, and skiing can often trigger or worsen symptoms. This is particularly frustrating for patients who take up these activities with high hopes of reducing their symptoms. One young woman recently reported that she tried one exercise after another in an attempt to relieve stress. At one point she was engaging in some kind of exercise every day—riding many miles on her bicycle, taking workout classes, jogging on an indoor track—and her symptoms kept getting worse. "I'm thin, trim, and strong," she said, "but I live with constant pain."

If TMJ sufferers take special care to consciously keep the teeth apart, exercise can be enjoyable and possibly beneficial to TMJ as well. However, the artificial method of keeping the teeth apart with tissue or cotton is inappropriate—even dangerous—during exercise.

Some patients have said that they are able to walk briskly and consciously keep their upper and lower teeth from touching. Brisk walking is an excellent conditioning exercise, and many people find it relaxing as well. Some people can jog and still keep their teeth apart, but most runners say this is difficult.

When people decide to get treatment for TMJ, one of the rewards is the ability to take up activities that once triggered or worsened their symptoms. Once treatment eliminates the cause of the problem, the person can use strenuous exercise for any desired reason—pleasure, stress management, weight reduction—without causing painful symptoms.

Some people who suffer from frequent mild to moderate headaches and neck and shoulder stiffness may find that relaxation techniques are sometimes helpful in preventing the onset of symptoms. Some people are more vulnerable to the effects of stress than others, and keeping stress levels low and manageable may help.

Most TMJ patients report that severity and frequency of symptoms rise and fall with changes in stress. Other patients report that symptoms apparently have nothing to do with stress. This area of health care still needs much exploration, and it's difficult to measure how stress affects conditions like TMJ.

Sometimes attempts to prevent or relieve symptoms can become a vicious self-defeating cycle, and the person in pain ends up full of self-blame and a sense of failure. The effort to relieve stress and practice good self-care techniques can become an enormous stress in itself.

Vickie Green was a patient whose life became a cycle of self-care and stress management that dominated all of her daily life. She had a rigid routine that she had developed over several years of trying to avoid pain.

Ms. Green often woke up with a mild headache, but even if she didn't, she took a long hot shower using a pulsating shower head to simulate massage. "If I had a headache, the long shower helped keep it from getting worse," she said. "If I didn't have one, I hoped the shower would prevent it. I stayed in the shower long enough to feel like a prune."

Ms. Green also played a relaxation tape before she left for work in the morning, was scrupulous about her diet, drank only herbal teas, and had long since given up cigarettes and any drink containing caffeine. "I watched every single thing I put in my mouth and ate a minimum of six times a day. I ended up avoiding certain restaurants because I didn't want any added sugar or food with preservatives," she said. "I had been told that low blood sugar could cause my headaches, or preservatives, or too much sugar, or even other people's cigarette smoke, so it was difficult to socialize with people and go places that are a normal part of life.

Ms. Green played another progressive relaxation tape in the women's lounge at her office during her lunch hour. Two or three times a week, she had a massage after work; other nights she took yoga classes. When she came home, she stood in a hot shower again and played still another relaxation tape when she went to bed.

Much of what Ms. Green did in her self-care program constitutes a healthful lifestyle. No health care practitioner would discourage any of these things in and of themselves. "If this regimen had worked all the time, I may have just kept it up for the rest of my life. But after three or four years of this, I still have pain." The cycle of stress management and pain prevention had left this patient unable to have a meaningful social life. Those few people still left in her life saw this regimen as neurotic, and she herself was sick of the self-absorption.

Ms. Green's case may sound unusual, but it isn't. I've heard this kind of story over and over again. Another patient, Joe Sterling, had a similar self-care regimen, which included regular visits with a hypnotist and meditation classes. If he skipped one of his classes or hypnosis sessions, he ended up filled with self-defeat. He ended up blaming his pain on his own inability to deal with what most people would consider normal stresses of life.

These examples aren't meant to discourage anyone from pursuing a healthful lifestyle. In fact, patients should engage in any activity that enhances their lives and contributes to their overall well-being. But in Ms. Green's case, she practiced the activities so obsessively and rigidly that they *prevented* her from living a "real" life. Mr. Sterling ended up deeply depressed because he thought he was too weak to handle life.

Because of cases like those described, bear in mind that self-help measures do not always work for TMJ sufferers. And even when they do, they should not necessarily be viewed as a substitute for treatment, especially when the measures themselves lead to self-absorption, depression, and excessively rigid living.

HEAT AND COLD

Once symptoms begin, there is one home remedy that can sometimes break the muscle-spasm cycle and relieve symptoms. Although this method is not used in my office treatment protocol, it is sometimes used by pain clinics and physical therapists. It is a practical method to use at home.

This method alternates the use of heat and cold therapy. The goal of the combination of heat and cold therapy is to irritate the muscle thermally in an attempt to break the spasm cycles. Anyone trying this method should use moist heat and ice alternately—hot packs for twenty minutes, cold packs for twenty minutes, nothing for twenty minutes. This hourly sequence can be repeated as needed.

Although it is less effective and penetrating, sometimes dry heat will accomplish what moist heat can. If wrapping hot moist towels around the head and neck is impractical, then a heating pad can be used. Sometimes using heat or cold alone will relieve muscle-spasm pain.

People have to decide for themselves at what point TMJ symptoms are manageable and at what point they are seriously interfering with their lives. This is an individual decision, but when life becomes an endless cycle of preventing symptoms or coping with them, seeking help is probably advisable.

16
A Call for Cooperation

My life was almost destroyed by this.
—a 51-year-old lab technician

*Again and again I was told there was no reason for the pain
and that it must be caused by psychological problems.*
—a 24-year-old medical student

*The problem has caused me more anguish than anything else
in my life—and to think there's been no need to suffer all this
pain for so many years.*   —a 33-year-old homemaker

*After years of searching, I'm furious that TMJ was missed
and the diagnoses I was given were so far off.*
—a 60-year-old fire fighter

Why is TMJ missed over and over again? Why
have so many people suffered needlessly? Why have TMJ
sufferers been forced to cope with little more than pain
relievers, often ineffective, and in many cases mind-altering
and addictive? These are frustrating questions that illustrate problems plaguing the health care community today.
   Almost every patient finally led to TMJ diagnosis and
treatment has had extensive work-ups and testing by
members of nearly all branches of the healing arts, from
physicians to nutrition counselors. Many have had these
work-ups more than once, as they sought help from one
practitioner then another. And, in retrospect, many people
are angry and frustrated because their conditions remained
unchanged no matter what therapies they tried. Because

they didn't understand the reasons for their suffering many were frightened by the pain.

Unfortunately, the TMJ treatment dilemma is complex. And the reason for the dilemma is rooted in the structure of the current health care delivery system. The healing arts, as we know them today, encompass various disciplines, including acupuncture, medicine, massage therapy, naprapathy, nutrition, physical therapy, osteopathy, dentistry, psychiatry, and psychology.

INBREEDING

For the most part, each branch tends to operate autonomously. Furthermore, in many cases health practitioners refuse to call upon—or they even outright reject—some premises of the other branches of health care. Because of this, each field tends to develop in an inbred fashion. Practitioners and researchers who reach outside their own fields and expand their knowledge are rare.

There are logical reasons for this situation. The amount of new material that must be regularly absorbed, simply to keep up with one's own field, is enormous. This makes it even more difficult to move outside a particular area of expertise and interest.

In addition, each branch of the healing professions has its own organizational structure and, regrettably, these structures seldom get along well with each other. Organizational structure does have its advantages. Each branch can focus on its own developments and trends.

However, the disadvantages of the existing structure block most interdisciplinary communication. This leads to an atmosphere where each branch is studying and learning independently and along its own philosophy of healing. As a result, information from differing branches of health care tends to be overlooked and, in many cases, even scorned.

Within each philosophical group, information is shared and lines of communication are more open. Members tend to refer patients to members within different specialties of the same branch. Physicians refer to other physicians. Osteopaths refer to other osteopaths. This kind of communication is routine. However, there are some exceptional clinicians who recognize the contributions other disciplines have made. These individuals think cross-referral is often in the best interests of the patient.

But, for the most part, there is little meaningful and coordinated communication between the various healing disciplines to work harmoniously on a patient's problems. Coordinated communication would allow two or more members of different branches of health care to come together to evaluate a patient and reach a diagnosis and treatment plan, while giving each appropriate approach individual and equal attention. An unfortunate lack of respect often exists among the groups.

THE RESULT: DISASTER

This situation has proved disastrous for TMJ sufferers. Often people wonder why TMJ was missed in the diagnostic processes they went through with various clinicians. But "missed" isn't exactly the way to describe it. Most physicians, for example, were not taught to recognize TMJ. Therefore it isn't on their lists of possible causes for headaches. You can't really miss what you didn't know about or understand in the first place. There is a definite need to bridge the information gap between all clinicians.

TMJ is not currently a separate specialty in dentistry. There are currently no comprehensive training programs for studying it. The various approaches used in the past have had mixed results, and the time allotted to studying the problem in dental school is scanty or nonexistent. Dental students are usually told the condition exists, but few are taught how to evaluate it, let alone treat it. Patients are still surprised when a dentist asks questions about TMJ symptoms during the course of a routine exam.

In medicine, the standard diagnostic approach is a procedure called differential diagnosis. When evaluating a patient, the physician lists (either mentally or in writing) the possible problems that may cause the symptoms the patient describes. To reach a proper diagnosis, the physician compares the characteristics of each of the listed diseases with the characteristics of the patient's condition. Diseases that do not match are eliminated.

In the course of diagnosing a patient complaining of headaches, this list will typically include, among other things, tumor, concussion, infection, and high blood pressure. Any one of these can cause headaches. But for the majority of patients, the causes of headaches can be limited to vascular headaches such as migraines or sinus disorders, and muscle-contraction or tension headaches. Of these types, migraine, sinus-related, and other vascular headaches make up the minority of all headaches. The majority of all headaches are muscle-contraction headaches, and the most frequent cause of these is TMJ. Unfortunately, this information isn't widely known, and is not included in training programs for clinicians.

AN ENLIGHTENED SYSTEM

If all health care practitioners were aware of TMJ, it would be high on the list of causes for this kind of chronic pain. If they also knew how to screen for TMJ (a procedure taking minutes), a patient could be advised to have this condition investigated.

In an enlightened health care system, patients who suffer from chronic headaches and other TMJ symptoms would be evaluated using knowledge from all the healing arts. Using this integrated concept, practitioners could untangle and interpret the mystery of the patient's symptoms and devise an appropriate treatment plan by considering many ideas. This would be the best way to avoid leaving patients in chronic pain because the experts whose help they seek lack information.

Once open dialogue is created and information is shared, more and more people will receive competent and prompt treatment for TMJ. When this dialogue is established, it may open the door to more discussion in other areas of health care. The people who study and treat TMJ may become pioneers in significantly integrating the knowledge and tools of all the healing arts. We will hear fewer stories of destroyed families, careers, and entire lives. We will reduce the number of patients who, when they finally seek evaluation for TMJ, consider it their last hope.

Questions and Answers

Here are questions people have asked me over and over again. It's my hope that the answers will clarify your understanding of TMJ.

Is there such a thing as a TMJ profile or a typical TMJ sufferer?
This is a common question, perhaps intended to narrow the field of sufferers. The typical TMJ sufferer usually has headaches. Beyond this, it's impossible to be specific.

Is it true that the majority of people who suffer from the symptoms of TMJ, and headaches in general, are women?
It is true that in the popular literature that discusses headaches, the majority of sufferers are women. The typical headache sufferer depicted in advertisements for headache pain relievers is usually a woman. However, headaches and other symptoms of TMJ seem to be fairly evenly distributed between the sexes. The majority of patients in my practice are women, but the majority of patients in almost all dental or medical practices tend to be women.

Women seem to know they need regular medical visits such as gynecological checkups and breast exams, and they make sure they get them. Women also tend to go to their dentists for routine checkups. In my experience, men more often wait until something is wrong. To treat dental problems that, because of neglect, have become emergencies, I see many more men than women.

There is still a kind of macho image that many men feel they must live up to. Men will deny pain more often than women. It's as if they see pain as something to be ashamed of.

I have heard of women complaining of a backache—a possible symptom of TMJ—and when no cause is found, they are labeled neurotic. Have you heard of men who suffer from backaches? What we usually hear is, "I threw my back out." (He might also attribute it to doing something "macho" like lifting a heavy object.) There is still pressure on men to disassociate themselves from conditions that have for too long been linked with the so-called weaker sex.

Does any one age group appear to be affected by TMJ problems more than others?

I've treated patients as young as ten and as old as seventy-eight. However, the bulk of my patients are in the prime of life, ages thirty to fifty. People wonder why, if a tooth-gearing problem exists, symptoms didn't begin in the stressful period of adolescence. While it's unknown why this disorder seems to strike in the middle years, certain diseases and disorders are common in childhood, others are common in older people. Perhaps TMJ will be found to be a disorder common to those in their prime. Perhaps it is simply related to the changes in the topography of the teeth—wearing down, more tooth replacement, and so forth. It may also be that the most active years are when we're more susceptible to traumas of the head and neck, which can trigger the problem. We can only hope that more research will reveal the answer to this question.

Do certain racial or ethnic groups tend to have higher incidence of TMJ than others?

Certainly none that we know of. TMJ appears to be about evenly distributed.

Is it common to have only middle-ear symptoms, but no headaches, neck stiffness, or any other common symptoms?

This isn't common, but it happens occasionally. If you are told that nothing is wrong with your ears, then TMJ would be a logical condition to investigate. But when starting the search for help, those with only middle-ear symptoms should begin with medical specialists, and TMJ should be among the last conditions to investigate.

My doctor says TMJ doesn't exist. Is this a common attitude among physicians?

It is more common than it should be, but few physicians deny the existence of TMJ. Rather, they might deny the high incidence of the condition, and doubt that it could be the major cause of headaches. Physicians have said it was hard to believe that all that pain could be caused by muscle spasms, especially small muscles like the external pterygoids.

Once TMJ is included on the list of possible causes for headaches, and training programs for all the healing arts are changed, patients will begin to be screened in physicians' offices for this problem. Physicians can be TMJ sufferers too, and if you ask such physicians whether they believe in the condition, you will hear no denials. *Anyone* who has ever been afflicted and then relieved of chronic pain caused by TMJ becomes a fast believer.

My dentist says the label of TMJ is being put on too many people, and that it's actually quite rare. Why is there such a vast difference of opinion?

Dentists not trained in TMJ might hear this message from someone they respect. Because they respect this individual, they may take the message seriously and absorb it as if it were truth. A dentist may hear the stories of a dentist who began to treat TMJ but had poor results. Many times, when treatment for TMJ fails, a judgment will be made that the condition probably wasn't TMJ in the first place. Knowledge of and belief in any concept often have more to do with exposure, training, and experience, either one's own or that of colleagues, than with the actual existence of a particular problem.

One dentist said I have TMJ. Another said I don't. Should I seek another opinion? Could I be a borderline case?

Dentists vary in their knowledge of the field. A "borderline case" is one in which the diagnosis is in question. Perhaps the patient isn't symptomatic, or suffers from symptoms mild enough that treatment isn't indicated at that time. Whenever there is a question it is always best to seek a second knowledgeable opinion.

I believe I have TMJ. I suffer from all the symptoms, and my dentist says I have a tooth-gearing problem. But I've spent a lot of time and money in pain clinics learning how to rise above the pain and live with it. I'm afraid to begin a new kind of treatment for fear that I'll lose the ability to cope with pain. Does this make sense?

It is certainly understandable that people are concerned about repeated disappointments in therapy. At times, learning to cope with pain seems like the most comfortable solution. However, in a case like this one, the person should have an evaluation for TMJ by a dentist who has a track record of successful treatment. If such treatment is available, the patient should go ahead with it. If someone had put a nail in your arm ten years ago and no one knew how to remove the nail, would you still keep the nail there when you have been shown that new nail-removing techniques have become available? Most people want to get rid of pain, not just cope with it. The techniques pain clinics use are wonderful in situations where no cause or cure can be found. There are other pain syndromes besides TMJ, and these clinics have helped many people live more normal lives.

I once had a bout with many of the symptoms of TMJ. It lasted about six months, and then it gradually went away and never came back. If I have the predisposition to TMJ, am I a "condition waiting to happen"?

You probably are. When you became symptomatic, your threshold or tolerance dropped, and when it went up, the symptoms went away. Any person with such an episode should keep TMJ in mind if these symptoms ever recur, or be mindful of the problem if restorative dentistry is ever needed. Remember, extensive dental work provided without knowledge of this problem can trigger TMJ.

Why do some people with a tooth-gearing problem become symptomatic, while others with the same problem remain symptom-free?

We don't know why some people are susceptible and others are not. We don't know why some people seem to be more susceptible to having muscles in the head and neck go into spasm. In the symptomatic person, we aren't sure why the susceptibility varies from week to week, day to day, and even year to year. We don't know why the tolerance threshold drops and symptoms occur. The severity of the tooth-gearing problem seems to have little to do with the severity of symptoms.

My therapist says I grind my teeth at night because of psychological conflicts. He says that when I work out my problems, my aching jaws and headaches will go away. If I have a tooth-gearing problem, how will correcting psychological problems help?

In a broad sense, solving psychological problems has little effect on TMJ. Any effect is over a very long time, and the tooth-gearing problem and, therefore, the potential to trigger the symptoms remains. We know that grinding or gnashing of teeth is one way humans—and other animals—manifest stress. We can see this when a dog feels threatened or is protecting its territory. So teeth grinding, or bruxism, as it is called, may be a psychological phenomenom. However, the physiological problem—the incorrect gearing of the teeth—is not. TMJ treatment addresses the gearing problem.

Psychotherapy is recommended when a patient is under extreme stress and is handling it poorly, or when underlying problems are preventing a person from functioning normally. Since TMJ is a physiological problem that is in no way brought on by psychological problems, it is most important to correct the tooth-gearing problem. Therapy can't correct a mechanical problem like TMJ.

I see a chiropractor regularly, and my back problems have greatly improved. However, while my headaches are better right after a visit, they always come back. Why?

People with back, neck, and shoulder problems and headaches commonly see practitioners such as massage therapists, osteopaths, naprapaths, and chiropractors. They often receive symptomatic relief for certain problems such as headaches, but nothing is done to permanently correct the tooth-gearing problem. They receive temporary relief because the therapies relax the muscles temporarily and break the spasms. However, because the causative reason has not been addressed, the spasms quickly start again. TMJ treatment corrects the problem that triggers the cycle of spasm and pain.

You seem to disapprove of drugs for anything. Are you against using drugs in health care in general?

It often must appear that I am against using pain-relieving drugs in general because I don't use them in treating TMJ. Actually, pain relievers can be valuable in numerous situations, including dentistry. I wouldn't want to drill teeth without using anasthesia. And medications of all kinds make modern medical care possible. What is inappropriate is the use of drugs in place of finding a reason for pain, for example, as the only therapy for chronic headaches when TMJ hasn't been explored. Too many patients are barely able to get through a simple interview because their bodies and minds are numbed with medication. Very often, the pain wasn't numbed, but the patient had lost the ability to care about it—or anything else in life. Sometimes patients don't even care that they don't care. This is the kind of drug therapy I'm opposed to.

I have dentures, but I also have TMJ symptoms. How can I have a tooth-gearing problem if I don't have my own teeth?

Many of my patients have dentures. A few have the dentures in the first place because they were told it would cure their TMJ. Unfortunately, removal of the teeth doesn't break the muscle spasms. If the spasms are present when the dentures are fabricated, they will be made in the same pattern as the original teeth, which caused the problem in the first place. TMJ treatment should break the muscle spasms and allow the jaw to reposition itself before adjustments are made to the dentures or new ones fabricated. A symptomatic patient should not have all his or her teeth removed as an initial treatment for TMJ. It rarely, if ever, corrects the problem, leaving the patient a "dental cripple."

If pain medications are rarely effective in treating TMJ patients, why do so many patients continue to take them?

People in chronic pain are frightened and depressed. They may at times feel as if they would try anything to help themselves. Sometimes the medications make them care about or notice the pain a little less than without them.

If I seek help for TMJ, I may need help with weaning myself from the drugs I have been taking for ten years. Is this often a difficult process for TMJ patients?

In general, I haven't found this to be a difficult problem. Most of my patients are more psychologically addicted than physically addicted. When they no longer have pain, they are usually glad to break the dependency. However, in some cases where the addiction is physical, or where dependency is established, patients are referred to physicians who can help them with this part of treatment. This is seldom a difficult phase of treatment.

Does TMJ run in families?

It is not documented, as it is for migraine, that TMJ runs in families. However, about 80 percent of the population has the predisposition for TMJ, and therefore it would appear logical that a familial connection will be found.

I have a very sensitive gag reflex, and I can't stand to have any foreign objects in my mouth. Would a nonremovable splint be appropriate in a case like mine?

In a case such as yours, I would generally use a nonremovable splint. However, using this type of splint involves slightly more risk and is much more costly.

I have migraines that are manageable with medications. I also have low blood sugar and often get headaches when I don't watch my diet. I also have premenstrual headaches and appear to be chemically sensitive. But, no matter what I change in my lifestyle, I still end up with headaches that seem to come and go for no reason. How would I find out if some of these headaches are TMJ related?

A TMJ evaluation would indicate whether you have a predisposition to the problem. There well may be a TMJ component, as it's not unusual to have numerous types of headache triggers. The TMJ treatment is like peeling away layers of an onion. When the TMJ component is removed, the patient can continue to evaluate other reasons for the pain. Often, once the TMJ-related headaches are gone, the total number of headaches from other causes may be significantly reduced.

My symptoms began after I was injured in an automobile

accident. I was once told that I have a predisposition to TMJ. Is it possible that my symptoms would never have been triggered if I hadn't been in that accident?

Yes. Many people go through an entire lifetime with a predisposition to TMJ and never become symptomatic. However, trauma can jerk or pull the muscles, creating a situation where it is easy for them to go into spasm. Again, we do not know why the majority of people with a predisposition to TMJ will never become symptomatic. But we do know that injury often triggers the symptoms.

My daughter's headaches began after she had orthodontic treatment. Why?

Teeth may not gear properly within the requirements of the jaw for many reasons—nature, the way the jaw grows, the way a person sleeps, dental work, injury, orthodontics, and dentures. If the teeth don't gear properly, the patient is always subject to TMJ. Sometimes orthodontics, as in this case, will create a gearing problem. Sometimes orthodontics are part of Phase II treatment, usually to get the teeth closer to correct gearing, so we can do an equilibration to complete the proper gearing on a minute level.

Does bruxism automatically indicate TMJ?

No. Bruxism is the body's attempt to even out discrepancies in the teeth. The basic gearing problem may create the muscle spasms, and it may create bruxing. Not all people with a gearing problem brux, and not all people with a gearing problem experience painful muscle spasms. We don't know why certain people will begin to brux, and we don't know why this bruxing will trigger painful symptoms. So, not all people who brux will have TMJ symptoms.

Is bruxing the same as a gearing problem?

Bruxing, or tooth grinding, is the *result* of a gearing problem in certain susceptible people. Often, the teeth that are causing the interference are avoided, and the other teeth are worn down. It's also important to remember that a person with a severe gearing problem may or may not have TMJ symptoms, and may or may not brux. Bruxism is both a cause and a symptom of the problem.

Will equilibration damage or weaken the teeth?

Equilibration on natural teeth most often involves working on the elevations of the teeth. This is advantageous because the enamel coating is usually thicker on the elevated portions of the teeth, and thinner in the "pits." Therefore equilibration rarely damages or weakens a tooth. Occasionally a patient will report increased sensitivity in a tooth that has been worked on. Whenever possible, we try to work within and on the fillings, inlays, and crowns. Sometimes we damage these and then must go in and replace them, However, there is seldom damage to the structure of a healthy natural tooth.

Will I be worse off if the TMJ treatment doesn't work?

One of the advantages of Phase I treatment, as described in this book, is that it can be stopped at any time, usually without any alterations in the patient's mouth. The patient can be left in the same condition as before treatment started. In this sense, a patient is certainly not worse off.

Unfortunately, many people seek TMJ treatment after having had orthodontia, surgery, or equilibrations before their symptoms were relieved. The rationale is that the alterations are needed in order for symptoms to be relieved. This is faulty thinking for the vast majority of cases. Until the jaw has relaxed into its normal position and the muscles are out of spasm, correcting the tooth-gearing problem is chancy. Some people luck out, and their symptoms go away when definitive treatment is done first, but the chances are slim.

I had mysterious tooth pain that was treated with several root canals. I began grinding my teeth after the work was done. Did I develop a tooth-gearing problem?

It is entirely possible that a tooth-gearing problem caused the tooth pain in the first place. On the other hand, you may have had solid reasons to have the root canals done—the teeth may have actually been dying. Once the root canals were done, you may have started to grind unconsciously in order to correct a gearing problem exacerbated or possibly even created by the dental work. It's impossible to look back and gauge the exact sequence of events. People with undiagnosable tooth pain or a bruxing habit should have TMJ screening.

I have had several bouts with TMJ symptoms, and have had TMJ diagnosed by two dentists. The treatment for my symptoms has been physical therapy. It has been quite effective, and whenever my symptoms flare up, I go for treatments. Is this maintenance therapy? If so, what's wrong with it?

Since TMJ has been diagnosed twice, we'll assume that you indeed have the condition. The periodic treatments you have sound like maintenance therapies in that they help you in the short run, but after a period of time the symptoms return, sending you back to the physical therapist. There is nothing wrong with this in and of itself. If this were the only solution to your problem, then it would be just fine, and if you were in severe pain, a true lifesaver. However, it is possible that you could be helped permanently, that your symptoms could go away and not return. The underlying problem can be corrected in the vast majority of cases. In the long run I don't see that permanent treatment is any more costly in money, lost time, and personal frustration than maintenace therapies. However, seeking a permanent solution for TMJ is a personal choice, and if you feel satisfied with the care you are getting, then by all means, continue it.

I have ground my teeth down to about half their original size by bruxing. How would you accomplish treatment in a case like mine?

Phase I of treatment would be the standard therapy described in this book. Phase II would involve correcting the tooth-gearing problem permanently, and if the teeth are severely worn down, it would most likely include reconstructive dentistry. We would need to rebuild what we call the "vertical dimension," the distance between the chin and the nose, which is determined by the length of the teeth when the jaw is closed. Remember that the jaw is basically a hinge and can be stopped in any position. People who have no teeth and do not wear dentures have a much shorter distance between the chin and the nose than those with teeth of normal size for them. When the teeth are worn down, we estimate the correct vertical dimension and build up the teeth, using plastic crowns, until we have established the most normal gearing pattern possible. The temporary crowns are then replaced with permanent ones.

My mother began having neck and shoulder problems at about age seventy. Lately she has been complaining of headaches, too. Is it common for a person to become symptomatic at such a late time of life? Has she had TMJ all her life, but is just symptomatic now?

There is no way to say for sure that your mother's headaches and other symptoms are caused by TMJ in the first place. It is important to begin by ruling out all other reasons for the pain. If no other reason is found for the symptoms, then TMJ would be a logical condition to investigate.

Only rarely do patients seek a TMJ evaluation after becoming symptomatic in their later years. In these few patients, it is likely that dental work has triggered the onset of symptoms. Often people have spent years wearing their teeth down, have old fillings, or have just become denture wearers for the first time. There's no way of knowing whether they were free of TMJ before their severe symptoms started. Because certain kinds of complaints—headaches, stiff shoulders, neck aches—are considered normal, a person won't even report them unless they are debilitating or beginning to be a regular occurrence.

Older people are more likely to have true joint derangement than younger people. Arthritis in the joint and problems with the disc aren't unusual either in older people. After all, an older person has spent years using his or her jaws. No matter what the signs and symptoms, it should always be determined whether the muscles are in spasm before assuming that surgery is the answer for pain around the joint.

I recently visited a headache clinic where I was given many tests and evaluations. However, TMJ was not considered. Would you recommend that TMJ be considered before I start other treatment?

Absolutely! You may or may not have TMJ. It is important to have TMJ included in *any* evaluation for the cause of headaches. Eventually, TMJ will be on the list of possible, and common, reasons for headaches. It is possible that you have more than one kind of headache. It is also possible that treatment suggested for you is *symptomatic* treatment, not a plan that treats the cause of the headaches you are experiencing. Any clinic that specializes in headaches should consider all causes. That can be said unequivocally.

Are you against people with TMJ taking stress-management courses, or learning meditation, or having regular massages? Aren't these things good for all people, regardless of whether they have a pain syndrome?

The things you mention are definitely good for people whether or not they have TMJ, migraines, high blood pressure, or even a bad cold. There is absolutely nothing wrong with any of these courses, techniques, or philosophies. People who have absolutely no symptoms of any disease or disorder can benefit from stress management, massage, and similar care. Many people find they are more productive when they schedule time for relaxation, play, spiritual growth, and exercise. Patients who are taking care of themselves in many ways often reenter normal life much more easily than those who lack hobbies, social lives, satisfying exercise programs, or even well-balanced diets.

What is disturbing is that so many people have been lured into taking up many of these practices as a way to manage TMJ. Sometimes the management therapies work in the short run. Sometimes they make a semblance of normal life possible for people who would otherwise walk around in severe pain practically every minute of the day. These therapies can't cure TMJ. TMJ is physiologically based; it is a tooth-gearing problem that causes muscle spasms in a susceptible person. No amount of relaxation therapy can correct a tooth-gearing problem.

The patients described in this book who have maintained a life, of sorts, by using these techniques were doing the best they could with the information they had. But when a patient seeks help for this problem and talks about life based on self-help, it is clear that, when carried to extremes, this life is stressful in itself.

When patients watch their diets so scrupulously because of their "allergies" that they can't go to restaurants with friends, when they are so afraid of their "hypoglycemia" that they feel obligated to carry food around with them and panic if they don't have it at the "right" time, or when they won't stay out past midnight on a Saturday night because it doesn't fit into their "program," then they are slaves to the stress management, diet, or whatever is supposed to be helping.them.

People who have never lived with pain probably think that those who live this way are rigid to excess. The people who live this way usually think so, too. Most people want to live within the mainstream of normal life.

When they are treated and their symptoms are gone, many patients keep some of the programs that have helped them. And why not? The programs are part of a healthful life that no health practitioner would discourage. But these people are also free to let go of practices they don't like or have observed or practiced to extremes.

I've been told my back pain is caused by my stressful lifestyle and that a certain amount of back pain is normal. I get occasional headaches, sometimes with the back pain and sometimes without it. Does this sound like TMJ?

An evaluation for TMJ is in order. The diagnosis implies that there is no systemic or structural reason for the pain. If TMJ is found to exist, treatment may eliminate spasms in the back muscles by treating other muscles in the chain.

Is TMJ treatment the same for all patients regardless of their symptoms? Is it true that patients with ear symptoms are treated with the same techniques as those with shoulder or back pain?

This is correct. TMJ treatment involves treating muscles in the head—specifically the external pterygoids. Remember: I don't *treat* "headaches" or "middle-ear problems." As a dentist, I treat tooth-gearing problems and muscle spasms. And as a dentist, I don't treat back muscles specifically. The key muscles involved in most of the symptoms of TMJ are located in the mouth, an area that dentists can legitimately treat. This is important because patients shouldn't say they went to a dentist to have their bad backs treated. They went to a dentist to have the tooth-gearing problem, which caused their symptoms, corrected. The relief of these other problems happens in response to what I do with these key muscles.

If muscle-contraction headaches are the most common type of headache, why has so little research been done to find causes and treatment?

Headaches in general have not been the focus of large amounts of research. This is largely because headaches in and of themselves are not life-threatening and are considered normal. And since most people have headaches at least once in a while, headaches are considered a manageable disorder. Vascular headaches have been considered more "glamorous" than muscle-contraction headaches, and what research has been done has usually been concentrated on the "migraine-type" headache.

If research were to be done on TMJ headaches, it would be logical to try to discover what makes people susceptible to muscle spasms. If we knew this, we would be able to discover why some people with tooth-gearing problems never become symptomatic and why others do.

Are there any rare symptoms of TMJ?

Occasionally a patient will talk about having very dry eyes. It is rare enough not to be included in the list of major, or common, symptoms. Some people mention just the opposite—eyes that tear very easily. A few people believe they have sinus problems because they get a stuffy nose along with their headaches. When the tooth-gearing problem is gone, many people who reported the stuffy-nose symptom often never get any headaches again. Thus, the headaches were probably not sinus headaches, but rather a reaction some people have to TMJ headaches.

I started wearing an athletic mouth guard when I jog, and my symptoms have improved. Should I seek treatment anyway?

You should certainly have an evaluation for TMJ. Whether you need treatment depends on how severe the symptoms are and how you feel your life is affected. Some athletes find their symptoms are worse with the mouth guard. There isn't any way to predict who will get worse or better with mouth guards.

My doctor says TMJ is just another fad disease, and interest in it will die in a year or two. How would you respond?

I would agree that interest in TMJ is high right now. Many people who had no idea why they were in pain are discovering the true answer. However, the disease is certainly not a fad. It's been around a long time, most likely ever since humans started to walk around on two legs. As more and more people begin to get appropriate treatment, and the "horror stories" on the way to diagnosis become fewer, then public interest will drop. I certainly hope so, because that will mean more people are getting proper treatment for the disorder.

Index